ABC of
Imaging in Trauma

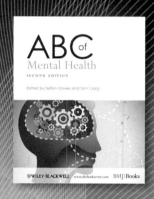
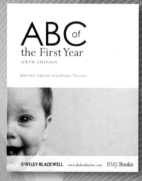
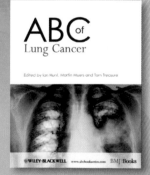
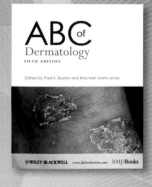
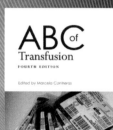
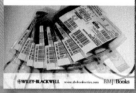
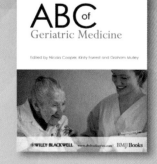

ABC of
Imaging
in Trauma

EDITED BY

Leonard J. King

Consultant Radiologist
Department of Radiology
Southampton University Hospitals NHS Trust
Southampton, Hampshire
UK

David C. Wherry

Professor of Surgery
Department of Surgery
Uniformed Services University of the Health Sciences
Bethesda, MD
USA

WILEY-BLACKWELL

A John Wiley & Sons, Ltd., Publication

BMJ|Books

This edition first published 2010, © 2010 by Blackwell Publishing Ltd

BMJ Books is an imprint of BMJ Publishing Group Limited, used under licence by Blackwell Publishing which was acquired by John Wiley & Sons in February 2007. Blackwell's publishing programme has been merged with Wiley's global Scientific, Technical and Medical business to form Wiley-Blackwell.

Registered office: John Wiley & Sons Ltd, The Atrium, Southern Gate, Chichester, West Sussex, PO19 8SQ, UK
Editorial offices: 9600 Garsington Road, Oxford, OX4 2DQ, UK
  The Atrium, Southern Gate, Chichester, West Sussex, PO19 8SQ, UK
  111 River Street, Hoboken, NJ 07030-5774, USA

For details of our global editorial offices, for customer services and for information about how to apply for permission to reuse the copyright material in this book please see our website at www.wiley.com/wiley-blackwell

Library of Congress Cataloging-in-Publication Data

ABC of imaging in trauma / edited by Leonard J. King and David C. Wherry.
    p. ; cm.
  Includes index.
  ISBN 978-1-4051-8332-1
1. Wounds and injuries–Imaging.   I. King, Leonard J.   II. Wherry, David.
  [DNLM: 1. Wounds and Injuries–diagnosis.   2. Diagnostic Imaging.   3. Emergencies.   WO 700 A1334 2010]
  RD93.7.A23 2010
  617.1′0754–dc22
                                                            2009013378

ISBN 978-1-4051-8332-1

A catalogue record for this book is available from the British Library.

Set in 9.25 on 12 pt Minion by Toppan Best-set Premedia Limited
Printed and bound in Malaysia by KHL Printing Co Sdn Bhd

1   2010

Contents

List of Contributors

Muaaze Ahmad, MB ChB FRCR
Consultant Radiologist
The Royal London Hospital
Whitechapel
London
UK

Simon Barker, MB ChB FRCP FRCR
Consultant Neuroradiologist
Wessex Neurological Centre
Southampton General Hospital
Southampton, Hampshire
UK

Antonio Belli, MD FRCS FRCS(SN)
Senior Lecturer in Neurosurgery
Division of Clinical Neurosciences
University of Southampton
Southampton, Hampshire
UK

Clare L. Bent, MB BCh FRCR
Interventional Radiology Fellow
The Royal London Hospital
Whitechapel
London
UK

Mark P. Bernstein, MD
Assistant Professor of Radiology
Trauma and Emergency Radiology
NYU Medical Center/Bellevue Hospital
New York, NY
USA

Gavin Bowyer, MChir FRCS(Orth)
Consultant Orthopaedic Surgeon
Southampton University Hospitals NHS Trust
Southampton, Hampshire
UK

**Mark W. Bowyer, MD FACS DMCC Colonel
(Ret) USAF MC**
Professor of Surgery
Chief, Division of Trauma and Combat Surgery
Director of Surgical Simulation
The Norman M. Rich Department of Surgery
Uniformed Services University of the Health Sciences
Bethesda, MD
USA

Christopher Burns, MD LCMDR USN MC
Surgical Resident
National Naval Medical Center
Bethesda, MD
USA

Xzabia Caliste, MD
Surgical Resident
Department of Trauma and Acute Care Surgery
Washington Hospital Center
Washington, DC
USA

Howard Champion, LRCP MRCS DMCC FRCS
Professor of Surgery and Senior Adviser in Trauma
Uniformed Services University of the Health Sciences
Bethesda, MD
USA

Catherine Cord-Uday, MBBS FRACS(Paed Surg)
Consultant Surgeon
Flinders Medical Centre
Bedford Park
Adelaide, SA
Australia

Evan Davies, BM FRCS Ed(Tr & Orth)
Consultant Orthopaedic Surgeon
Southampton University Hospitals NHS Trust
Southampton, Hampshire
UK

David Elias, MBBS BSc MRCP FRCR
Consultant Musculoskeletal Radiologist
Department of Diagnostic Imaging
King's College Hospital NHS Foundation Trust
London
UK

Peter K. Ellis, MB BCh MRCP FRCR FFRRCSI
Consultant Radiologist
Royal Victoria Hospital
Belfast, Northern Ireland
UK

Sivadas Ganeshalingam, MA MBBS FRCS FRCR
Radiology Fellow
The Royal London Hospital
Whitechapel
London
UK

David Gay, MB BS FRCR
Fellow in Musculoskeletal Radiology
Nuffield Orthopaedic Centre
Oxford, Oxfordshire
UK

Iain Gibb (Lieutenant Colonel), MB ChB FRCS FRCR RAMC
Consultant Radiologist and Army Consultant Advisor in Radiology
Royal Hospital Haslar
Gosport, Hampshire
UK

Mark Griffiths, MRCP FRCR
Consultant Radiologist
Southampton University Hospitals NHS Trust
Southampton, Hampshire
UK

Leonard J. King, MB ChB FRCP FRCR
Consultant Radiologist
Department of Radiology
Southampton University Hospitals NHS Trust
Southampton, Hampshire
UK

Graham Lloyd-Jones, BA MBBS MRCP FRCR
Specialist Registrar in Radiology
Southampton University Hospitals NHS Trust
Southampton, Hampshire
UK

Jason H. M. Macdonald, MB BS MRCP FRCR
Specialist Registrar in Neuroradiology
Wessex Neurological Centre
Southampton General Hospital
Southampton, Hampshire
UK

Matthew B. Matson, MRCP FRCR
Consultant Interventional Radiologist
Royal London Hospital
Whitechapel
London
UK

Niall Power, MRCPI FRCR
Consultant Radiologist
St Bartholomew's and The Royal London Hospitals
London
UK

Anne G. Rizzo, MD FACS
Associate Professor of Surgery
Virginia Commonwealth University School of Medicine
Richmond, VA
USA; *and*
Uniformed Services University of the Health Sciences
Bethesda, MD
USA

James Ryan, OstJ MCh FRCS DMCC FFAEM(Hon)
Emeritus Professor of Conflict Recovery
University College London and St George's University of London
London, UK; *and*
International Professor of Surgery
Uniformed Services University of the Health Sciences
Bethesda, MD
USA

Madeleine Sampson, MB ChB FRCP FRCR
Consultant Radiologist
Southampton University Hospitals NHS Trust
Southampton, Hampshire
UK

Richard A. Schaefer, MD MPH DMCC COL MC USA
Associate Professor of Surgery
Chief, Division of Orthopaedic Surgery
Norman M. Rich Department of Surgery
Uniformed Services University of the Health Sciences
Bethesda, MD
USA

James H. Street, MD
Department of Trauma and Acute Care Surgery
Washington Hospital Center
Washington, DC
USA

James Teh, MB BS BSc MRCP FRCR
Consultant Musculoskeletal Radiologist
Nuffield Orthopaedic Centre
Oxford, Oxfordshire
UK

Ioannis Vlahos, BSc MBBS MRCP FRCR
Consultant Thoracic Radiologist
St George's NHS Trust
London, UK; *and*
Assistant Professor
New York University
New York, NY
USA

David C. Wherry, MD FACS FRCS LRCP DMCC
Professor of Surgery
Uniformed Services University of the Health Sciences
Bethesda, MD
USA

Foreword

Some four decades ago, as a recently qualified doctor, I managed victims of trauma without the benefit of trauma systems, without well tried management protocols and without today's imaging technology. Digital imaging did not exist and "urgent" X-ray films were often still wet from the chemical processor, making interpretation less than optimal. Computed tomography and magnetic resonance imaging were still prototypes or on the physicist's drawing board and ultrasound scanning was in its infancy. Digital, whole-body scanners, such as the Lodox Statscanner, were something approaching science fiction. In the intervening period between then and now, trauma care, like many other aspects of medicine, has progressed immeasurably, as has the part played by imaging technology and techniques.

It is incumbent on all who provide emergency, in-hospital trauma care to be aware of the current range of diagnostic and therapeutic techniques that radiology and radiologists bring to the management of trauma. This short, but comprehensive book, the *ABC of Imaging in Trauma*, will do exactly that.

After reading this book, medical personnel will have an understanding of current imaging concepts *and* their clinical relevance, a point well made by the book's editors in their introductory chapter. They also go on to point out that the fundamental goals of imaging are assisting staff in quickly identifying the range and severity of injuries and, where possible, intervening to arrest life-threatening haemorrhage. They also endorse the point: imaging techniques are there to complement clinical skills and acumen, not to replace them.

The fundamental aim of this book is to act as a practical guide on the scope and interpretation of emergency imaging procedures used in assessing the severely injured. It more than achieves this in a host of ways, the more outstanding being: the key points summary boxes at the beginning of each chapter; discussion of relevant clinical and demographic information before going on to discuss imaging techniques; and the richness and quality of the illustrations and line diagrams. These factors also add to the ease of finding relevant information.

It is of some import that the last four chapters of this book cover paediatric trauma, imaging trauma in pregnancy, ballistics and blast injury and imaging of major incidents and mass casualty situations. Managing trauma in children and pregnant women can be particularly trying. This book provides a systematic review and excellent short guide to imaging techniques in both situations. Major incidents are now almost commonplace. Knowledge of the role of imaging in casualty triage in such incidents, is one key to saving lives. This book provides that knowledge.

Those who become victims of severe trauma, whether civilian or military, will have the best outcome if cared for by experienced, multidisciplinary teams working to well-tried protocols. One of these protocols is what this excellent book is about: a guide to the place of the many forms of imaging available in trauma management algorithms.

All who are interested in, or have a role in hospital-based trauma care, should read this book. It will make them better carers.

My own anticipation is that the next edition will be even better.

P. Roberts, CBE MS FRCS
Professor of Military Surgery Emeritus
Royal College of Surgeons of England
December 2009

Acknowledgements

The editors would like to thank Professor Norman Rich and the Department of Surgery at the Uniformed Services University of Health Sciences, Bethesda, Maryland, for their assistance in the production of this book, and Dr Graham Lloyd-Jones for his assistance in the production of illustrations.

CHAPTER 1

Introduction

Leonard J. King[1] and David C. Wherry[2]

[1]Southampton University Hospitals NHS Trust, Southampton, Hampshire, UK
[2]Uniformed Services University of the Health Sciences, Bethesda, MD, USA

Trauma is a leading cause of morbidity and mortality in the developed world, accounting for 39 deaths per 100 000 population in the United States in 2005 and around 800 000 deaths per year in Europe. Deaths resulting from trauma typically follow a tri-modal distribution (Figure 1.1). The first peak, which accounts for 50% of all trauma deaths, occurs within the first few minutes after injury. Very few of these victims can be salvaged and thus prevention is the key to significantly decreasing the rate of immediate deaths. The second peak occurs from a few minutes up to several hours after injury, often due to uncontrolled bleeding, and accounts for 30% of trauma-related mortalities. With appropriate medical care many of these patients can be saved by prompt identification and management of correctable injuries. The last peak occurs days to weeks after the injury. Outcome during this period of late deaths depends in part on how cases are managed in the preceding periods.

Recognition that trauma care was previously fragmented and disorganized with poor outcomes has helped to stimulate innovations in trauma care including trained paramedics, advanced trauma life support (ATLS) training for surgeons and in-house response teams in many hospitals. These developments, supported by technological advances including imaging techniques, have led to an improvement in the quality of emergency care. Nevertheless, motor vehicular collisions, domestic and industrial accidents, assaults, gunshot wounds and injuries related to acts of terrorism continue to challenge the management of trauma by medical teams throughout the world.

During the hospital phase of resuscitation, modern technology and medical facilities should complement the physician's clinical skills to improve decision making for trauma patients. There are a number of different imaging modalities that can be used to assist in the management of these patients, each with a variety of strengths and weaknesses. Plain radiographs remain a useful tool, particularly for the assessment of limb fractures and dislocations. In recent years, however, there have been significant developments in the imaging of major trauma, particularly with the introduction of multidetector computed tomography (MDCT), which allows rapid acquisition of detailed whole body cross-sectional imaging.

Coupled with advances in post-processing techniques, MDCT now also allows the routine application of computer-generated high-quality multiplaner reformat (MPR) and three-dimensional volume-rendered images in addition to the axial plane images (Figure 1.2). This new technology has redefined the role of plain radiographs, ultrasound and computed tomography in the evaluation of victims of major trauma. At institutions where the full range of diagnostic imaging facilities are readily available, whole body MDCT has become the imaging investigation of choice in stable patients following the initial ATLS recommended trauma series (chest, lateral cervical spine and pelvis). Some trauma centres are also fortunate enough to have CT within the emergency department and are advocating CT for all but the most unstable trauma patients, a policy which is not suitable for many other hospitals where CT facilities are remote from the resuscitation area or may not be immediately available for an unstable trauma patient. In such circumstances and in more austere situations, alternative imaging strategies will need to be employed, including additional plain radiographs, ultrasound, intravenous urography and on-table in-theatre angiography.

Ultrasound has been used in the investigation of abdominal trauma since the 1970s and interest grew in the 1990s with the availability of hand-held ultrasound machines and the development of the limited focused assessment of sonography in trauma (FAST) technique (Figure 1.3). The FAST technique enables non-radiologists with limited training to perform a rapid ultrasound examination in the resuscitation room looking for free intraperitoneal fluid (Figure 1.4) with a reasonable degree of accuracy. FAST can be used to triage a haemodynamically unstable patient with significant free fluid to surgery; however, the absence of free fluid does not exclude a significant intra-abdominal injury requiring surgical intervention. Even in the hands of experienced observers the sensitivity of ultrasound for demonstrating organ lacerations and mesenteric or retroperitoneal injury is poor and thus it cannot be routinely used to exclude injury as a stand-alone technique. Where facilities are limited and no CT is available, a policy of admission for observation and repeat ultrasound by an experienced operator can be used but should not be considered best practice.

Imaging findings in conjunction with clinical assessment can be crucial in providing the critical information required to make key management decisions. Thus, an understanding of current trauma

ABC of Imaging in Trauma. By Leonard J. King and David C. Wherry
Published 2010 by Blackwell Publishing

imaging concepts and their clinical relevance is essential for all medical personnel involved in the immediate hospital care of trauma patients whose outcome may depend on rapid assessment of the nature and severity of their injuries, allowing appropriate medical management and surgical and non-surgical intervention.

Although the precise role of imaging and the choice of modality will vary depending on the clinical scenario and the availability of equipment and local expertise, the fundamental goals remain the same – that is, assisting clinical staff in rapidly identifying the range and severity of injuries in the trauma patient and, where possible, intervening to arrest life-threatening haemorrhage with use of endovascular procedures. It is important for those involved in trauma care to recognize the place of imaging in relation to other clinical activities and how it fits into the clinical algorithm. The ATLS approach in trauma care is summarized in Box 1.1.

Although there are helpful published criteria for determining the need for cranial and cervical CT scanning following trauma, there are as yet no universally accepted criteria for determining when whole body CT is indicated, and local policies will vary. Most patients are triaged to CT on the basis of mechanism of injury, such as a high-velocity motor vehicle collision, and an initial clinical assessment indicating significant injury, particularly where there is evidence of two or more anatomically remote injuries, for example head injury plus a pelvic fracture or chest injury plus femoral fracture, etc. Whole body CT is also helpful in assessing patients with clinical signs of external trauma in whom the mechanism of injury is unknown, for example a patient found unconscious with bruising, lacerations or an obvious fracture and no available witness statement.

The purpose of this book is to provide a concise and practical guide to the role, performance and interpretation of emergency imaging procedures in patients with major trauma, such as those encountered in road traffic accidents, major disasters such as earthquakes and the victims of civilian or military conflict. The author-

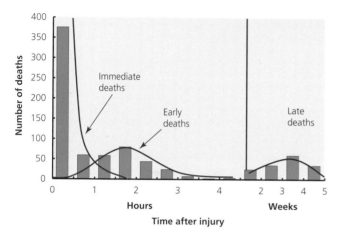

Figure 1.1 Graph illustrating the trimodal distribution of deaths following trauma. Graph taken from the ATLS Manual, 2005. Reproduced with the permission of the American College of Surgeons.

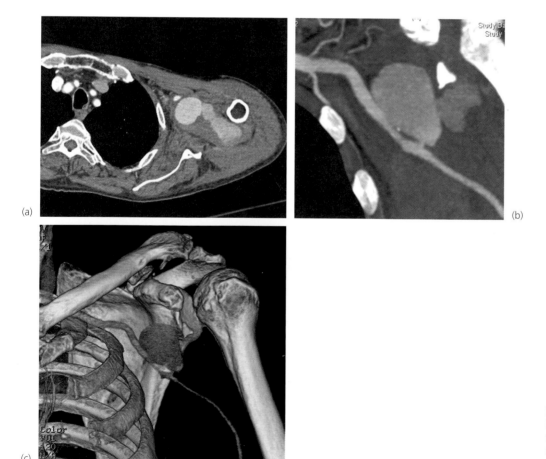

(a)

(b)

(c)

Figure 1.2 (a) Conventional axial images; (b) coronal multiplaner reformat; and (c) 3D volume-rendered CT images of a traumatic axillary artery pseudoaneurysm.

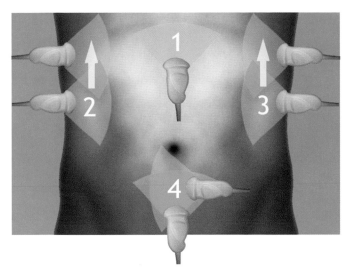

Figure 1.3 Ultrasound probe positions for a limited focused assessment of sonography in trauma ultrasound examination.

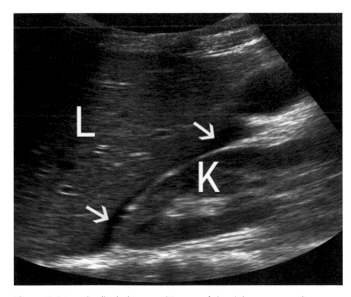

Figure 1.4 Longitudinal ultrasound image of the right upper quadrant demonstrating a small volume of free intraperitoneal fluid (arrows) between the liver (L) and the right kidney (K).

Box 1.1 **ATLS approach in trauma care**

A Primary survey and assessment of ABCDEs
  1 Airway with cervical spine protection
  2 Breathing
  3 Circulation with control of haemorrhage
  4 Disability: brief neurologic evaluation
  5 Exposure/Environment: undress patient and prevent hypothermia
B Resuscitation
  1 Oxygenation and ventilation
  2 Shock management – IV fluids
  3 Management of life-threatening problems identified in the primary survey
C Adjuncts to primary survey and resuscitation
  1 Monitoring
    a Arterial blood gases
    b Ventilation
    c End tidal CO_2
    d Electrocardiogram
    e Pulse oximetry
    f Blood pressure
  2 Urinary catheter and nasogastric tube placement
  3 Radiographic and other diagnostic studies
    a Chest x-ray
    b Pelvis x-ray
    c Cervical spine x-ray (lateral)
    d FAST or DPL
D Secondary survey: total patient evaluation
  1 Head and skull
  2 Maxillofacial and intra-oral
  3 Neck
  4 Chest
  5 Abdomen (including back)
  6 Perineum/rectum/vagina
  7 Extremities
E Adjuncts to the secondary survey (performed after life-threatening injuries have been identified and managed)
  1 Computed tomography
  2 Contrast studies
  3 Extremity radiographs
  4 Endoscopy and ultrasonography
F Definitive care

ship draws on a large number of experienced radiologists and surgeons who manage trauma in their daily practice, both in civilian and military settings. The boundaries of these two seemingly separate spheres are becoming increasingly blurred. Civilian casualties from ballistic trauma and acts of terrorism are frequently encountered in cities throughout the world and lessons learned from medical care in military conflict have relevance in rural, urban and suburban non-military settings.

CHAPTER 2

Head and Neck Trauma

Simon Barker[1], Jason H. M. Macdonald[1] and Antonio Belli[2]

[1]Southampton General Hospital, Southampton, Hampshire, UK
[2]University of Southampton, Southampton, Hampshire, UK

OVERVIEW

- Rapid diagnosis and management of primary intracranial injuries will help limit secondary injuries
- Rapid access to computed tomography (CT) scanning is required for all patients with a significant head injury
- Patients who deteriorate after CT scanning require repeat scanning
- If undertaking urgent initial CT scanning of the head, the cervical spine should also be scanned

---

Head injury

Trauma is the most common cause of death and permanent disability in the first few decades of life, and head injury is responsible for the majority of this morbidity and mortality. About 1.4 milllion head injuries occur in the United Kingdom each year; 270–313 individuals per 100 000 population are admitted to hospital with this diagnosis per year, and the mortality rate is 6–10 per 100 000 population per year. Death is four times more common in males than females. Road traffic accidents account for a significant proportion of head injury fatalities. Falls represent a higher percentage of injuries at the extremes of life.

Plain radiographs have no primary role in the management of patients with head injury. Computed tomography (CT) is now widely available, fast and accurate in the detection of intracranial haemorrhage. Magnetic resonance scanning is more sensitive for the detection of parenchymal abnormalities, but longer examination times, difficulties in monitoring patients and lower sensitivity for diagnosing fractures have limited its use in primary diagnosis. Boxes 2.1 and 2.2 provide indications for CT in head injury.

Head injuries may be classified as primary or secondary lesions. Primary lesions are a direct result of the traumatic force, which may be penetrating (projectile) or non-penetrating (blunt). In the United Kingdom, blunt injury remains the most common mechanism. Shear-strain deformation of neurones or blood vessels due to rotational acceleration of the head is the commonest mechanism

---

Box 2.1 **Indications for CT scanning in adult head injury**

Immediate CT (within 1 hour of request)
- GCS <13 when assessed in Emergency Department
- GCS <15 two hours after Emergency Department assessment
- Suspected open or depressed fracture
- Signs of basal skull fracture
- Seizure
- Focal neurological deficit
- More than one episode of vomiting
- Anticoagulant therapy or coagulopathy, plus if any amnesia or loss of consciousness since the injury

CT within 8 hours
- Pre-traumatic amnesia >30 minutes
- Age >65 years if any amnesia or loss of consciousness since the injury
- Dangerous mechanism, plus if any amnesia or loss of consciousness since the injury (e.g. pedestrian or cyclist hit by motor vehicle; ejected vehicle occupant; fall >1 m or 5 stairs)

Box 2.2 **Indications for CT scanning in paediatric head injury**

- Age <1 year; GCS <15 on assessment in Emergency Department (Paediatric GCS)
- Age <1 year; bruise, or swelling or >5 cm scalp laceration
- Dangerous mechanism (high-speed RTA, fall >3 m, high-speed projectile injury)
- Suspected non-accidental injury
- Witnessed loss of consciousness >5 minutes
- Seizure (with no history of epilepsy)
- Suspicion of open or depressed fracture
- Tense fontanelle
- Signs of basal skull fracture
- Focal neurological deficit
- Amnesia (antegrade or retrograde) >5 minutes
- Abnormal drowsiness
- Three or more discrete episodes of vomiting

---

of primary intra-axial injuries. Localized fracture or in-bending of the skull may cause direct injury to the underlying brain.

Secondary lesions develop as a result of primary intracranial lesions or as the neurological effects of systemic injuries. Box 2.3 lists the primary and secondary lesions.

ABC of Imaging in Trauma. By Leonard J. King and David C. Wherry
Published 2010 by Blackwell Publishing

Box 2.3 **Classification of head injuries**

Primary lesions
Skull fracture
Extra-axial haemorrhage
• Extradural haematoma
• Subdural haematoma
• Subarachnoid haemorrhage
Intra-axial injury
• Diffuse axonal injury
• Cortical contusion
• Subcortical grey matter injury
• Primary brainstem injury
• Intracerebral haematoma

Secondary lesions
Diffuse cerebral swelling
Hypoxic injury
Cerebral herniation
Traumatic territorial infarction

Skull fracture

Between 25 and 30% of severely injured patients have no identifiable skull fracture. Fractures (Figure 2.1) may be linear (more often associated with extradural and subdural haematomas), depressed (more often accompanied by local brain injury) or involve seperation of a cranial suture. Pneumocephalus may complicate skull-base fractures with a dural tear involving the paranasal sinuses, mastoid ear cells or middle ear.

Extradural haematoma

Laceration of the middle meningeal artery by a fracture is the usual cause of extradural haematoma (Figure 2.2). This is a relatively uncommon injury, but accounts for 10% of fatal head injuries. The temporoparietal region is the most common site. The haematomas are lentiform in shape, and on CT scanning two-thirds are hyperdense and one-third mixed density. Injury to a dural venous sinus by a fracture of the occipital, parietal or sphenoid bone is a much less common cause of extradural haematoma.

Subdural haematoma

Stretching and tearing of bridging cortical veins as they cross the subdural space is the usual cause of subdural haematoma (Figures 2.3 to 2.6). The arachnoid may also be torn, leading to a mixture of blood and cerebrospinal fluid in the subdural space. Subdural haematoma is seen in up to 30% of fatal head injuries. Acute subdural haematomas are crescentic in shape, and on CT, 60% are hyperdense and 40% mixed density. A subacute subdural haematoma will become isodense to cortex within a few days to weeks of the trauma. Chronic subdural haematomas are often loculated and have a lentiform or crescentic shape. They are predominantly hypodense on CT but may contain areas of fresh haemorrhage.

Traumatic subarachnoid haemorrhage

Subarachnoid haemorrhage (Figure 2.7) is seen scattered in superficial sulci and cerebrospinal fluid cisterns in most moderate to severe head injuries.

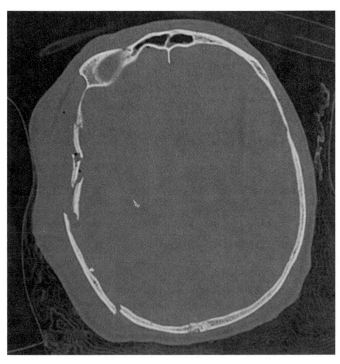

Figure 2.1 CT scan showing comminuted fracture of right skull vault.

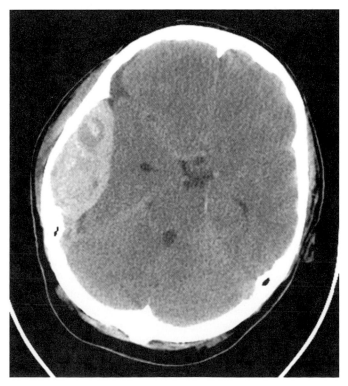

Figure 2.2 CT scan showing acute extradural haematoma over right temporal lobe. Note the lentiform shape.

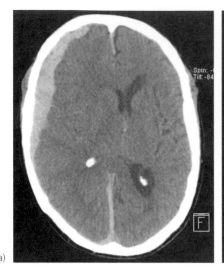

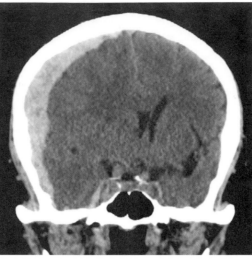

Figure 2.3 (a) Axial CT scan showing acute subdural haematoma over right cerebral convexity with midline shift of the brain to the left; (b) coronal reformat demonstrates the full extent of the haematoma and crescentic shape.

(a)

(b)

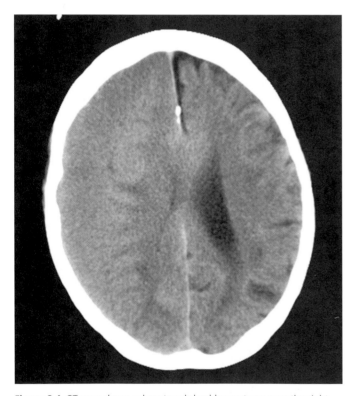

Figure 2.4 CT scan shows subacute subdural haematoma over the right cerebral hemisphere is of similar density to the cortex. Cortical sulci and the right lateral ventricle are effaced.

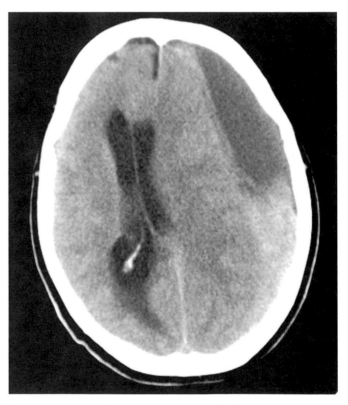

Figure 2.5 CT scan shows layering has occurred in this chronic subdural haematoma.

Diffuse axonal injury

Sudden deceleration and rotational forces on the brain cause axonal shearing injuries, which may be accompanied by laceration of adjacent capillaries. Diffuse axonal injury (DAI) (Figures 2.8 and 2.9) occurs most frequently at the grey/white matter interface, particularly in the fronto-temporal region. Lesions are also seen in the posterior corpus callosum. More severe injury involves the basal ganglia, thalamus and dorsolateral midbrain. As 80% of axonal shearing injuries are non-haemorrhagic, a CT scan is often normal. Haemorrhagic shearing injuries are seen as multiple small hyper-dense foci. DAI is typically associated with immediate loss of consciousness at the time of injury.

Cortical contusions

Cortical contusions (Figure 2.10) are bruises of the brain surface and occur in up to 45% of patients with non-penetrating head injuries. They are less frequently associated with initial loss of consciousness than DAI. They are caused by the brain striking a bony ridge or dural fold, and so occur in characteristic locations: 50% in the antero-inferior temporal lobes and 35% in the antero-inferior frontal lobes. Superior frontal parasagittal contusions are less common. Early CT scans may show only subtle low-density lesions or low-density lesions mixed with small hyperdense foci of haemorrhage. Later scans will show more and larger lesions than on initial CT, often with delayed haemorrhage.

Intracerebral haematoma

Intracerebral haematomas are caused by shear-strain injuries to intraparenchymal arteries or veins and may be difficult to distinguish from haemorrhagic contusion or DAI.

Subcortical grey matter and brainstem

Primary trauma to the thalamus, basal ganglia and brainstem represents less than 10% of primary traumatic brain injuries. Most injuries are due to disruption of small perforating blood vessels caused by shearing forces, although some are due to the brainstem striking the tentorial incisura. CT shows petechial haemorrhages in the affected brain.

Cerebral herniation

Bony ridges of the inner table of the skull and dural septa divide the cranial cavity into compartments. The capacity for expansion

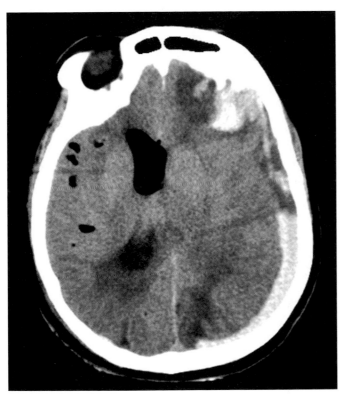

Figure 2.6 CT scan showing pneumocephalus. There is air (jet black) in the right frontal horn and right sylvian fissure, as well as left frontal contusion and mixed-density acute subdural haematoma on the left.

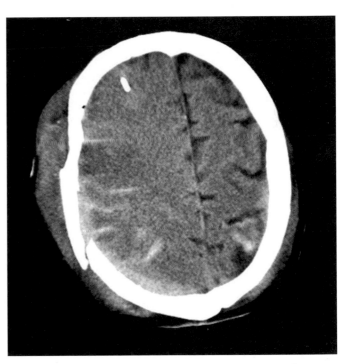

Figure 2.7 CT scan showing subarachnoid blood in the depths of sulci as well as a subdural haematoma underlying the fracture. An intracranial pressure monitor lies in the right frontal lobe.

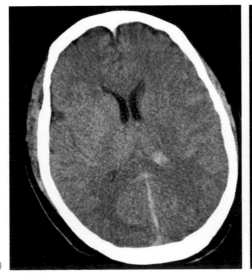
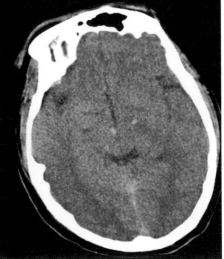

Figure 2.8 (a, b) CT scans showing haemorrhagic diffuse axonal injury. Small hyperdense foci are seen in the corpus callosum, midbrain, thalamus and internal capsule.

(a)

(b)

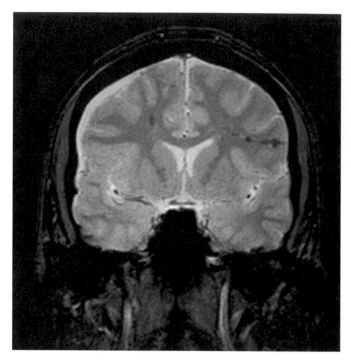

Figure 2.9 Magnetic resonance imaging: a coronal gradient echo T2 image shows a shallow subdural haematoma (bright) over the right cerebral convexity and haemorrhagic DAI as scattered low-signal (dark) foci in the frontal lobes.

Traumatic cerebral infarction

Traumatic cerebral infarction is usually due to brain displacement across dural surfaces; occipital lobe infarction is the most common and is due to compression of the posterior cerebral artery against the tentorial incisura by herniated temporal lobe.

Cerebral ischaemia

Marked changes in global or regional cerebral blood flow occur in many patients with Glasgow coma score ≤8 and some authors consider cerebral ischaemia to be the most important cause of secondary brain injury following severe head injury.

Diffuse brain swelling

One or both cerebral hemispheres may swell independently or in association with focal injuries. Diffuse cerebral swelling (Figure 2.11) is seen in 10–20% of severe head injuries and is more common in children.

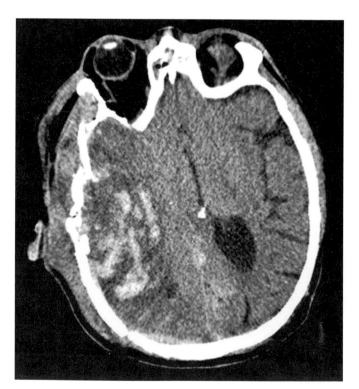

Figure 2.10 CT scan showing mixed density right temporal contusion.

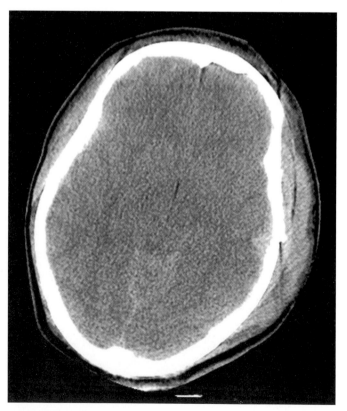

Figure 2.11 CT scan showing diffuse cerebral swelling. There is loss of normal differentiation between grey and white matter and effacement of cortical sulci, the third ventricle and basal cisterns.

of brain tissue without ill effect is very limited. Cerebral herniation is the displacement of brain tissue from one compartment to another and results in compression of the brain, cranial nerves and blood vessels (Box 2.4).

Vascular injury

Injury to cervical and intracranial arteries as a result of trauma is uncommon but is increasingly recognized with the advent of high-resolution scanning of these patients.

Relatively mild blunt trauma to the neck vessels may cause arterial dissection. In some patients dissection of the extracranial carotid or vertebral artery may remain asymptomatic and heal spontaneously, but in others there may be early or delayed distal embolization. The diagnosis can be made non-invasively with magnetic resonance angiography or CT angiography (Figure 2.12).

Penetrating injuries to the neck are more likely to cause pseudoaneurysm, arteriovenous fistula or vessel transection than blunt trauma. Facial vascular injuries usually follow penetrating trauma but may occur after blunt trauma if there are multiple fractures. Occlusion of external carotid vessels is probably asymptomatic in many blunt facial injuries because of the rich collateral circulation of the face.

Damage to intracranial arteries may result from blunt or penetrating trauma. Skull base fractures may cause petrous or cavernous carotid dissection or a direct carotid cavernous fistula (Figure 2.13).

In a direct carotid cavernous fistula there is arterial communication with the cavernous sinus, which may lead to reversal of flow in the ophthalmic veins with engorgement of the orbit, and reversal of flow in cortical veins with a risk of subarachnoid haemorrhage. The fistula is treated by endovascular obliteration. Intradural internal carotid artery dissections are rare, but have a poor prognosis because of the propensity for subarachnoid haemorrhage (Figure 2.14).

Non-vascular soft tissue neck injuries

Soft tissue neck trauma presents a considerable clinical challenge because of the multiple organ systems contained within a small volume of tissue. The anterior and lateral portions of the neck are most susceptible to injury, with the spine providing protection posteriorly. The neck is divided into three horizontal zones for clinical purposes. Zone I is bound inferiorly by the thoracic inlet and superiorly by the cricoid cartilage; zone II lies between the cricoid cartilage and the angle of the mandible; zone III lies between the angle of the mandible and the base of skull. The important anatomical contents of each zone are listed in Figure 2.15a. CT is

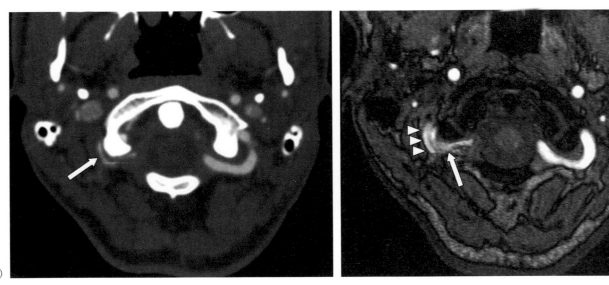

(a) (b)

Figure 2.12 Right vertebral artery dissection. (a) CT angiogram at the level of C1 vertebra shows small calibre of right vertebral artery lumen (arrow); (b) magnetic resonance angiogram at the same level shows bright intramural haematoma (arrowheads) as well as small vessel lumen (arrow).

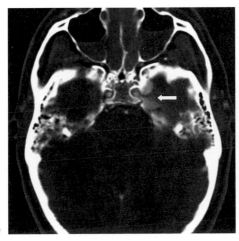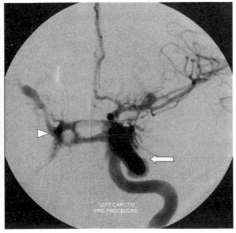

Figure 2.13 Left carotid cavernous fistula. (a) CT angiogram shows abnormal opacification of left cavernous sinus (arrow); (b) left internal carotid angiogram shows filling of enlarged left cavernous sinus (arrow) and of right cavernous sinus (arrowhead).

(a) (b)

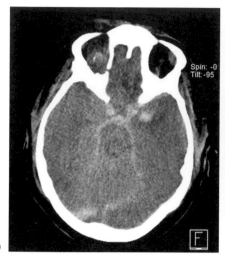

(a)

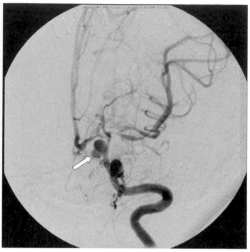

(b)

Figure 2.14 Traumatic supraclinoid carotid pseudoaneurysm. (a) CT scan demonstrates subarachnoid haemorrhage; (b) left internal carotid angiogram shows pseudoaneurysm (arrow).

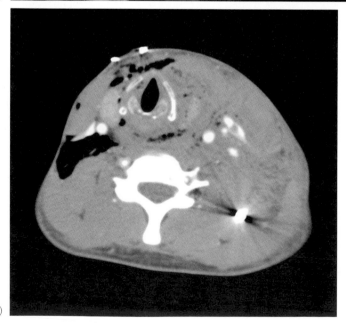

Internal carotid artery
External carotid artery
Vertebral artery
Facial nerve
Glossopharyngeal nerve
Hypoglossal nerve

Angle of mandible

Common carotid artery
Jugular vein
Phrenic nerve
Vagus nerve
Hypoglossal nerve
Tongue base
Pharynx
Larynx

Cricoid cartilage

Subclavian artery
Subclavian vein
Great vessels
Recurrent laryngeal nerve
Trachea
Oesophagus
Lung apex

(a)

(b)

Figure 2.15 Soft tissue neck injuries. (a) schematic diagram of the neck showing boundaries of zonal anatomy and important contents of each zone; (b) CT scan of neck after injury by improvised explosive device. Metal fragments are visible. There is extensive surgical emphysema and there has been left-sided vascular injury with associated haematoma.

mandatory for assessment of suspected injuries in this region (Figure 2.15b). Injuries in zone I are most likely to be clinically occult.

Facial fractures

Facial trauma is commonly seen after fights, falls and road traffic accidents. Injuries predominantly occur to the mid-face or mandible. Plain radiographs remain important in the initial assessment of facial trauma, but high-resolution CT scanning will often provide more useful information than the clinical examination and radiographs combined, and is increasingly used.

Mandibular fractures

These are common, exceeded only by nasal and zygomatic fractures in adults. The mandible is the strongest bone in the face but has points of weakness, which predispose to fractures; nearly 50% of fractures are bilateral.

Mid-face fractures

Nasal fractures

Isolated nasal fractures account for about 50% of facial fractures. They are diagnosed clinically or by a coned lateral radiograph.

Tripod fractures

Tripod fractures (Figure 2.16) are the second most common facial fractures after nasal bone injuries. The zygomatic arch, the frontal process of the zygoma, and the superior and lateral walls of the maxillary antrum are involved in this fracture.

Maxillary fractures

Maxillary fractures (Figure 2.17) are described by the Le Fort classification, although in practice the injuries are often not symmetrical and occur in combination. CT is required for their accurate diagnosis and management.

Le Fort I: a horizontal fracture that passes through the lower third of the nasal septum, medial and lateral walls of the maxillary sinus, and the pterygoid plates separating the hard palate and alveolar process from the mid-face.

Le Fort II: this is pyramidal in configuration with the apex at the lower part of the nasal bones. The fracture passes through the medial and inferior walls of the orbit, the lateral walls of the maxillary sinuses below the zygomatico-maxillary suture and extends posteriorly across the ptyergoid plates.

Le Fort III: the fracture passes through the nasal bones, posteriorly and laterally through the medial plus lateral walls of the orbit

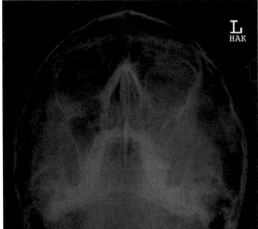
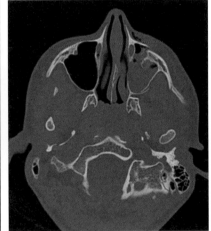

Figure 2.16 Left tripod fracture seen on (a) plain radiograph; (b) axial CT scan.

(a)

(b)

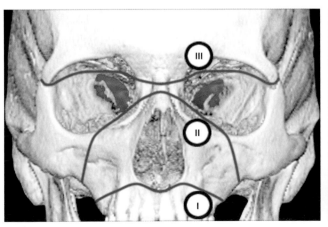
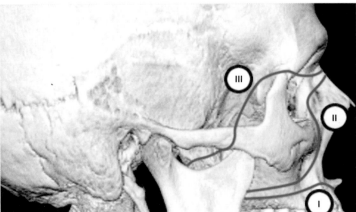

(a)

(b)

Figure 2.17 (a) Frontal and (b) lateral views of surface-rendered 3D reconstruction of CT scan with superimposed lines of fracture in Le Fort I, II, and III injuries.

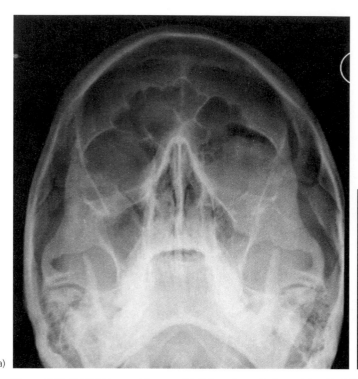

(a)

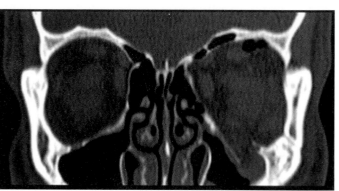

(b)

Figure 2.18 Orbital blow-out fracture. (a) Plain radiograph shows left orbital floor fracture with soft tissue opacification of upper maxillary antrum; (b) coronal CT scan shows herniation of orbital contents through fracture of orbital floor.

and the zygomatic arch, and extends through the posterior wall of the maxillary sinus to involve the ptyergoid plates, thus separating the entire mid-facial skeleton from the cranial base.

Orbital fractures

Orbital fractures may result from a direct blow to the orbit or as part of a mid-face injury. Blow-out fractures (Figure 2.18) are caused by non-penetrating trauma to the eyeball, with the force transmitted to the floor or medial wall of the orbit and the fracture fragment directed away from the bony orbit. They most commonly involve the orbital floor; orbital fat and/or inferior rectus muscle may herniate through the bony defect or become trapped by the fracture margins.

Upper third facial fractures (nasoethmoidal complex)

Upper third facial fractures are uncommon injuries often resulting from a severe blow over the bridge of the nose. The nasal bones, nasal septum, ethmoid bones including the cribriform plate, and the frontal sinuses may all be involved with attendant risks of cerebrospinal fluid rhinorrhoea and intracranial infection.

Further reading

National Institute for Health and Clinical Excellence. *Triage, assessment, investigation and early management of head injury in infants*, children and adults. Clinical guideline. September 2007 (www.nice.org.uk/CG56).

CHAPTER 3

Chest Trauma

Ioannis Vlahos[1] and Howard Champion[2]

[1]St George's NHS Trust, London, UK, *and* New York University, New York, NY, USA
[2]Uniformed Services University of the Health Sciences, Bethesda, MD, USA

OVERVIEW

- The supine anteroposterior radiograph is an important adjunct to the primary survey
- Pneumothorax may be occult on supine chest radiographs
- Contrast enhanced computed tomography (CT) gives a comprehensive and detailed examination of the thorax, including assessment of the thoracic aorta
- Multiplanar reformat images of chest CT scans should routinely be evaluated for aortic and diaphragmatic injuries, and fractures to the thoracic spine and sternum
- A mediastinal haematoma can arise from a range of thoracic injuries and is not diagnostic of aortic injury
- Tracheobronchial injury should be considered in the presence of a pneumothorax that is unresponsive to tube drainage

---

Introduction

Thoracic injury is common in major trauma. The thoracic cage provides a degree of protection to the cardiopulmonary system and the mediastinum. However, even in blunt force trauma, particularly in children where the thorax is compliant, the internal contents of the thorax may be injured without apparent bony injury. Therefore, the absence of significant osseous rib trauma does not preclude major internal injury.

The majority of thoracic injuries occur from blunt trauma rather than penetrating injury, and knowledge of mechanism of injury can aid the imaging evaluation. Specifically, the change in velocity (delta V) of a motor vehicle collision and knowledge of whether the occupant was restrained, ejected or required extraction alter the pre-test probability of significant injury and may influence the imaging interpretation.

Techniques

Chest radiography

The initial imaging evaluation of thoracic injury is usually with a chest radiograph. In major trauma this will usually be a portable

---

ABC of Imaging in Trauma. By Leonard J. King and David C. Wherry
Published 2010 by Blackwell Publishing

supine anteroposterior (AP) film. Slightly over-penetrated radiographs permit pleuroparenchymal evaluation plus simultaneous evaluation of the thoracic spine and paramediastinal planes (left paraortic, left and right paramediastinal lines). In minor trauma, erect departmental high kVp films are preferable, allowing better evaluation of the mediastinal contours and lung parenchyma.

Initial evaluation of radiographs should focus on the critical factors necessary for immediate patient management in an order comparable to the advanced trauma life support (ATLS) ABC system. A more detailed systematic comprehensive evaluation may then follow (Box 3.1).

On AP films the mediastinum may appear widened, the heart enlarged and fluid levels may be obscured. With penetrating injuries from gunshot wounds it can be useful to place a radio-opaque marker such as a paper clip on the entrance and exit wounds in order to estimate the bullet trajectory.

Ultrasound

Ultrasound can be used to assess the pleural and pericardial cavities for fluid usually as part of a focused assessment of sonography in trauma (FAST) scan. It can also be used to guide procedures such as placement of central lines or drains into pleural fluid collections.

Computed tomography (CT)

Computed tomography (CT) has revolutionized the evaluation of cardiothoracic trauma. Current generation multidetector CT (MDCT) scanners image the chest in a few seconds, giving a motion-free comprehensive evaluation of the entire thorax. CT improves the sensitivity, accuracy and confidence of injuries suggested by chest radiographs, as well as identifying and characterizing additional injuries that cannot be evaluated by plain films, including vascular, airway or pericardial injuries. CT also demonstrates subtle air or fluid collections in the pleural space and the course of penetrating injuries. Multiplanar reconstructions can be routinely used to evaluate the pulmonary parenchyma, mediastinum, diaphragm, spine and sternum in the coronal or sagittal plane. Intravenous contrast administration is essential for evaluation of the cardiomediastinum. A normal enhanced CT effectively excludes any significant thoracic injury with the possible exception of the rare instance of an isolated myocardial contusion without an associated pericardial effusion sternal, or mediastinal injury.

Chest wall and rib injury

Isolated rib, clavicular or scapular fractures may not be of major clinical significance but are indicative of the force and pattern of injury. Scapular blade fractures are associated with spine injuries in 25% of cases. Fractures of the upper three ribs indicate high-impact injury and are associated with vascular injuries in up to 10% of cases.

The extent of rib fractures is frequently underestimated by AP chest radiographs. CT accurately depicts fractures and in combination with advanced imaging techniques such as maximum intensity or volume-rendered projections simplifies visualization of the injuries. This is particularly helpful when evaluating flail segments in which four or more contiguous ribs are fractured in two places (Figure 3.1).

Sternal and sternoclavicular joint dissociations result from high-impact injuries and have recognized associations with cardiac or mediastinal injury. These injuries are usually inconspicuous on supine AP films and may be difficult to detect even on dedicated lateral sternal or oblique sternoclavicular projections. Sternal injuries may be difficult to appreciate even on CT, as they are frequently horizontally oriented. The presence of a substernal haematoma should prompt a careful review of the sternum, including sagittal reconstructions (Figure 3.2). Sternoclavicular or costovertebral dissociation injuries are easily appreciable at CT. Posterior dislocation of the clavicle in relation to the sternum is associated with mediastinal vascular, oesophageal and brachial plexus injuries.

Thoracic injury can be associated with a large chest wall or breast haematoma (Figure 3.3) containing significant volumes of blood, particularly when there are lacerations of multiple intercostal arteries, the internal mammary arteries or the periscapular vessels. This manifests on imaging as diffuse soft tissue swelling or a localized collection, and may demonstrate active contrast extravasation on CT.

Pulmonary injury

Lung injury is a common manifestation of blunt trauma. Parenchymal contusions are relatively common, representing areas of pulmonary haemorrhage and oedema. These are best evaluated by CT, typically appearing as areas of ill-defined non-segmental peripheral parenchymal consolidation, frequently adjacent to ribs or vertebrae against which the lung has been compressed. Air bronchograms are relatively rare as the peripheral bronchi are usually filled with blood. Contusion should be differentiated from atelectasis, which is common due to mucus plugging, prolonged supine positioning, pain or depressed consciousness-induced diaphragmatic splinting and aspiration. Pulmonary contusions are rarely apparent on chest radiographs within the first 1–2 hours of injury unless severe and extensive. Early air-space opacity on radiographs is thus more likely to reflect atelectasis or aspiration (Figures 3.4 and 3.5). At CT, contusion is differentiated from atelectasis or aspiration by its frequent non-dependent location, proximity to areas of impact and lack of segmental or fissural demarcation. The lung fissures pose no impediment to the transference of traumatic kinetic energy, whereas atelectasis and consolidation are constrained by the normal lobular and segmental bronchopulmonary anatomy (Figures 3.6 and 3.7).

Pulmonary lacerations are more significant injuries of the lung parenchyma that can occur with blunt trauma or more commonly following penetrating injury. They represent an interstitial tear with local haemorrhage plus an air leak, and there may be an associated pneumothorax (Figure 3.8). Lacerations may appear initially as simple contusions or as an ill-defined opacity with a central

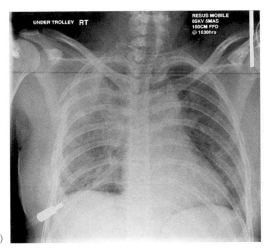
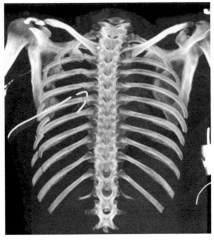

Figure 3.1 Blunt trauma from high-velocity vehicle collision. (a) Anteroposterior chest x-ray demonstrates multiple right-sided rib fractures with underlying consolidation due to contusion; (b) CT maximum intensity projection following chest drain insertion assists visualization of the rib fractures confirming a flail segment of the upper thorax.

(a)

(b)

Axial Sternal Fracture

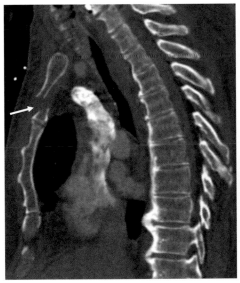
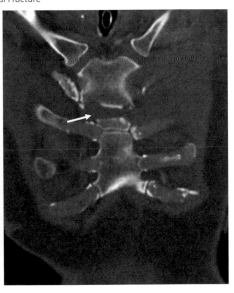

Figure 3.2 Horizontally oriented sternal fracture depicted on (a) sagittal and (b) coronal CT reformats (arrows). Note the retrosternal anterior mediastinal haematoma.

(a)

(b)

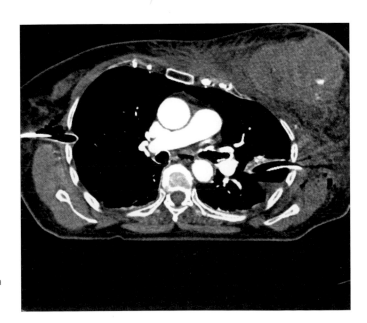

Figure 3.3 Left breast haematoma following blunt trauma. CT scan shows a large collection with active contrast extravasation, which was subsequently treated by internal mammary artery embolization

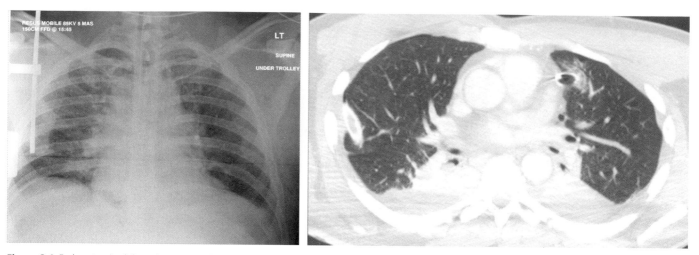

Figure 3.4 Early extensive bilateral symmetrical airspace opacity on chest x-ray post trauma suggestive of atelectasis and confirmed by segmental dependent distribution at CT. Note the intraparenchymal chest drains.

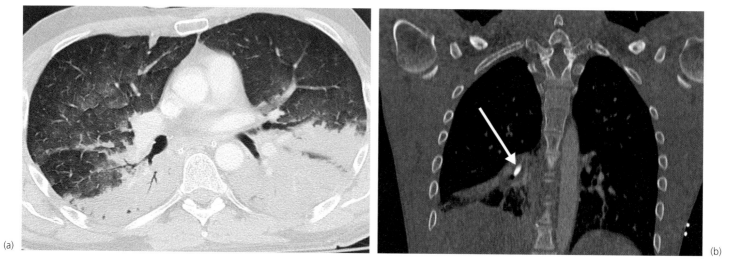

(a)

(b)

Figure 3.5 Two cases of trauma-related aspiration. (a) Dependent consolidation plus widespread ground glass opacity on axial CT following a near drowning; (b) right lower lobe collapse on a coronal CT reformal due to an aspirated tooth following facial injury (arrow).

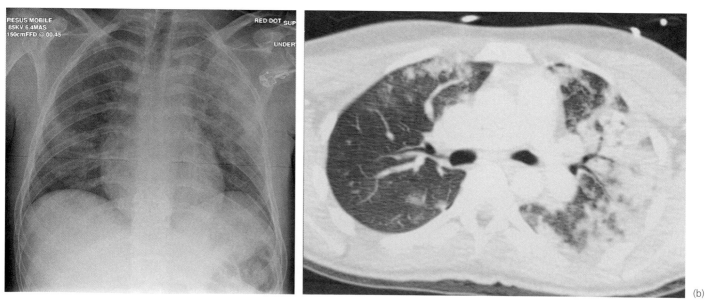

(a)

(b)

Figure 3.6 (a) Extensive asymmetric airspace opacity on chest x-ray following major trauma and delayed vehicular extraction; (b) CT scan confirms non-dependent, non-segmental airspace opacity not bounded by fissures or segmental anatomy consistent with contusion.

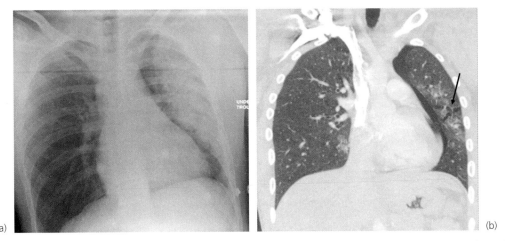

(a) (b)

Figure 3.7 Blunt force injury with extensive contusion on chest x-ray (a). Coronal CT scan reconstruction (b) reveals multiple linear lacerations in the lung parenchyma (arrow) and an associated pneumothorax.

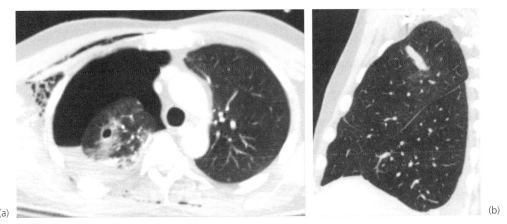

(a) (b)

Figure 3.8 Pulmonary laceration following stabbing. (a) Initial CT scan demonstrates ill-defined parenchymal air-space opacity due to contusion with a central focal lucency due to the laceration. An associated pneumothorax is present; (b) follow-up CT scan demonstrates infilling of a laceration tract by haematoma.

pneumatocele. The lesions subsequently fill in with serous fluid or haematoma, developing an air-fluid level or a solid mass. Resolution typically starts within days and completes over a period of weeks. Occasional persistence may cause suspicion of a solid or cavitary malignant pulmonary nodule if the initial traumatic event is not recalled.

Pleural injury

In supine patients, pneumothoraces collect in the anteroinferior pleural space and may not be visible on supine films. The only sign may be a thin lucency along the diaphragmatic or cardiac border without the conventional pleural edge seen in the lung apex on erect radiographs (Figure 3.9). As the anterior pneumothorax becomes larger, the normally acutely marginated costophrenic sulcus may become enlarged – the so-called "deep sulcus" sign. This is an indication of significant pressure exerted by the anterior pneumothorax and a sign of increasing tension. CT is more sensitive to the detection of small pneumothoraces and may identify unusual appearances such as subpulmonic or loculated pneumothoraces due to pleural adhesions (Figure 3.10).

Pleural fluid collections collect in the most dependent postero-inferior aspect of the thorax. On supine radiographs all causes of pleural fluid appear as a diffuse increase in density over a hemithorax without loss of visualization of the underlying vascular markings. The meniscus of a pleural fluid collection seen on erect films is frequently absent. A pleural collection resulting in increased opacity of a hemithorax must be distinguished from lung collapse or increased attenuation due to rotation or poor film centering. When the cause of increased opacity is technical, the increased density will extend throughout the ipsilateral soft tissues.

CT is sensitive to small pleural fluid collections and by Hounsfield unit (HU) measurement may differentiate between different causes of pleural fluid. Simple fluid collections may be reactive and measure 0–20 HU. Haemothorax initially measures >20–30 HU, although with time may separate into a lower attenuation superior layer and a denser dependent layer. Acute haemorrhage from intercostal vessels may occasionally be identified. Low-density pleural fluid (≤-10 HU) indicates fat suggestive of a chylothorax following thoracic duct penetrating injuries, either in the right posterior mediastinum or at its insertion into the confluence of the left internal jugular and subclavian veins.

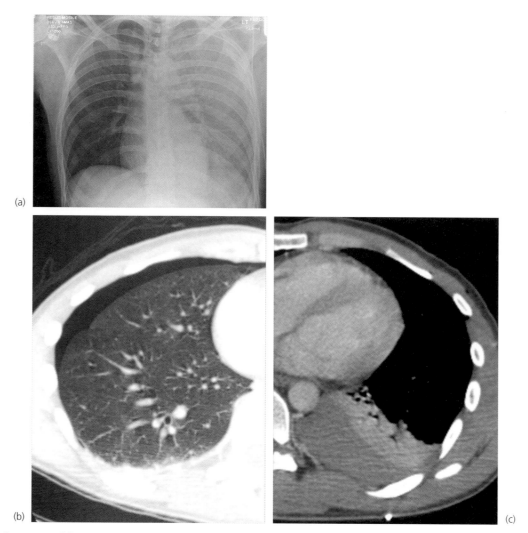

(a)

(b)

(c)

Figure 3.9 Blunt chest trauma following motor vehicle collision. (a) Chest x-ray demonstrates subtle right-sided peridiaphragmatic lucency secondary to a supine pneumothorax confirmed by (b) CT on lung windows; and (c) a left-sided supine haemothorax confirmed by a dependent hyperdense pleural fluid collection on mediastinal windows.

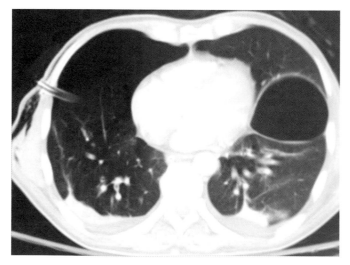

Figure 3.10 CT scan demonstrating a right anterior supine pneumothorax with an indwelling drain and an untreated loculated intrafissural left-sided pneumothorax that was not apparent on chest x-ray.

Drains should generally be sited in an anterior location for pneumothoraces and a posterobasilar location for pleural fluid collections. CT rapidly and accurately confirms intrapleural chest drain location and may exclude errant or suboptimal intra-fissural locations (Figure 3.11). Transparenchymal pulmonary chest drain tracts are not uncommon, resembling tubular parenchymal contusions or lacerations and resolving in a similar fashion.

Mediastinal injury

Traumatic disruption of the aorta is a potentially catastrophic injury, with 50% of patients expiring at the scene of injury or within the first hour of trauma. This is usually a deceleration injury, which rarely occurs at speeds of less than 30 mph. The predominant diagnostic sign is the presence of a mediastinal haematoma. Mediastinal widening on an AP supine radiograph may indicate haematoma, but is commonly due to mediastinal fat or vascular

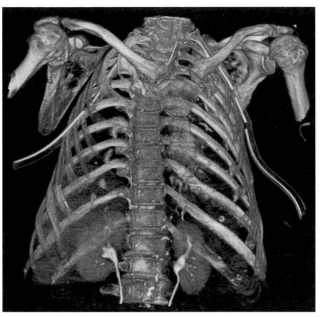
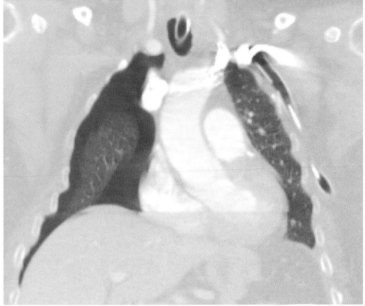

Figure 3.11 Bilateral chest drain placement for traumatic pneumothoraces. Volume-rendered CT and coronal reconstruction demonstrate that the left-sided drain lies in the chest wall outside the pleural space.

Box 3.2 **Plain film signs suggestive of traumatic aortic injury**

- Widened mediastinum
- Loss of clarity of the aortic contour
- Apical pleural haematoma (cap)
- 1st rib fracture
- Depression of left main bronchus
- Deviation of nasogastric tube to the right

---

ectasia in older patients. Loss of clarity of the superior mediastinal paraortic contours is supportive of a possible haematoma. Ancillary signs of aortic injury such as depression of the left main bronchus, a left apical pleural cap, rightward tracheo-oesophageal displacement and associated fractures of the first or second ribs may aid evaluation (Box 3.2).

Contrast-enhanced MDCT is currently the imaging gold standard for evaluation of mediastinal injury, enabling demonstration of a haematoma and the underlying aetiology. The majority of mediastinal haematomas are not due to aortic disruption. An anterior haematoma separated from the aortic arch by a compressed mediastinal fat plane is typically due to the rupture of small mediastinal veins or sternal injuries. Posterior mediastinal blood is usually secondary to spinal injuries (Figure 3.12).

At CT, aortic injury is invariably associated with haematoma but frequently demonstrates only minimal disruption to the aortic wall contour. This is usually just after the origin of the left subclavian artery, sited near to the ligamentum arteriosum (Figure 3.13). This is thought to be a relative point of anchoring of the aorta around which torsion forces are exerted. The term "traumatic dissection" is a misnomer, as true traumatic dissection rarely occurs.

The confirmation of aortic injury by conventional angiography is no longer routinely indicated due to the additional radiation exposure, intravenous contrast administration and time delay to operative management that this incurs.

A small minority of acute aortic disruptions may initially go unnoticed and a traumatic calcified pseudoaneurysm may form (Figure 3.14). Increasingly, both acute and chronic traumatic pseudoaneurysms are treated with endovascular metallic stent-grafts.

Cardiac and pericardial injury

Cardiac and pericardial injuries are relatively rare, and usually follow anterior chest wall injury, often with associated soft tissue bruising. Pericardial collections due to air, or more frequently haematoma, are readily identifiable on CT (Figure 3.15). Tamponade can be identified by evidence of compression of the right ventricle, dilation of the superior vena cava (SVC) and inferior vena cava (IVC), and by hepatic congestive changes. Larger pericardial collections can also be identified on FAST ultrasound by examining subcostally above the left lobe of the liver. Rupture of the pericardium can cause herniation of the heart and consequent pump failure.

Cardiac contusions predominantly affect the anterior wall of the right ventricle and can result in heart failure. Imaging may be unhelpful and the diagnosis relies on clinical suspicion, electrocardiogram (ECG) abnormalities and elevated cardiac enzymes, although there will usually be associated sternal, mediastinal or pericardial abnormalities. Myocardial disruption is usually the result of penetrating injury and is rarely imaged, as it is fatal unless contained by a tamponading pericardium. Right ventricle rupture following blunt trauma likewise has a poor prognosis and rupture

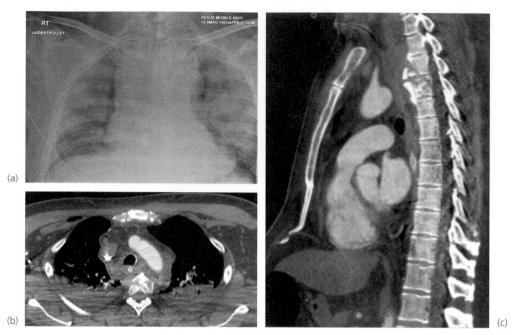

Figure 3.12 (a) Supine chest x-ray demonstrates significant mediastinal widening in a patient following a fall from 10 metres; (b) axial and (c) sagittal reformat CT images confirm a mediastinal haematoma which is centred over the posterior mediastinum related to spinal fractures.

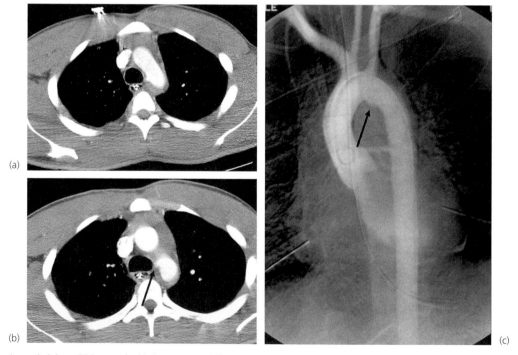

Figure 3.13 Traumatic aortic injury. CT images (a, b) demonstrate diffuse increased density of the mediastinum consistent with a haematoma centred around the aortic arch. There is a small aortic wall irregularity medially (arrow) just beyond the ligamentum. The aortic disruption is also depicted by catheter angiography (c) (arrow), although this is not usually necessary.

of the base of the aorta is instantly lethal. Conversely, a rupture of the right atrial appendage should be treatable. Rupture of the chordae tendinae and the cardiac valves can also occur.

Penetrating injury from a stab wound usually involves the right ventricle but is occasionally lateral enough to catch the left ventricle, and even more rarely the left anterior descending artery. Survival rates up to 50% have been reported and patients arriving with vital signs generally have a good prognosis, particularly if associated shock is related to tamponade as opposed to near exsanguination. Gunshot wounds to the heart produce multiple holes in

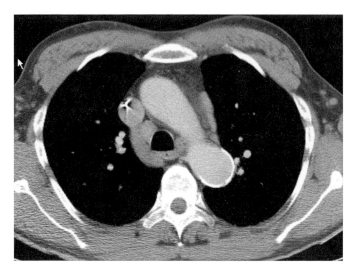

Figure 3.14 Chronic peripherally calcified aortic post-traumatic pseudoaneurysm typically arises in the region of the ligamentum arteriosum. Incidental mediastinal lymphadenopathy is also present.

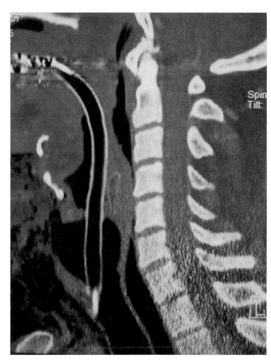

Figure 3.16 Proximal tracheal rupture following severe neck trauma from an attempted suicide. CT scan demonstrates loss of structural integrity of the trachea with associated surgical emphysema and air tracking into the superior mediastinum.

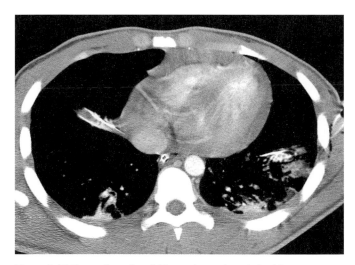

Figure 3.15 Traumatic pericardial haematoma characterized by a high-density fluid collection around the heart in a patient with extensive bilateral lower lobe contusions and sternal injury (not shown).

multiple chambers, sometimes with septal injury, and have a poor prognosis.

Tracheo-oesophageal injury

Tracheobronchial or oesophageal injuries are both very uncommon. In the cervical region they are usually the result of direct trauma (Figure 3.16). Within the thorax these injuries are usually the product of raised intrathoracic pressure or compression against the spine. Penetrating and iatrogenic injuries due to attempted intubation, nasogastric tube insertion or transoesophageal echocardiography can also occur (Figure 3.17).

Tracheobronchial injury occurs in less than 1% of major trauma. Most cases involve the distal 2.5 cm of the trachea and the proximal bronchi with a right-sided preponderance. The main feature of such injuries is the presence of marked pneumomediastinum and pneumothorax unresponsive to chest tube drainage. The lung may appear detached from the mediastinum – the "fallen lung" sign. Additional signs may include ectopic positioning of an endotracheal tube or hyperexpansion of the endotracheal tube cuff. Distal bronchial injury can also occur and may present late with persistant atelectasis.

Pneumomediastinum is a common feature on trauma films and may reflect rupture of an isolated adjacent sub-pleural pulmonary bleb, extension of a pneumothorax into the mediastinum or a tracheo-oesophageal injury. Pneumomediastinum can be differentiated from pneumopericardium by extension above the aortic arch and continuation over the diaphragmatic surfaces. The distinction is easier at CT, where smaller quantities of mediastinal air are detectable and associated injuries may be excluded. At CT, small mediastinal air bubbles may indicate the site of injury. Although frequently dramatic in appearance, both pneumomediastinum and pneumopericardium per se are rarely physiologically significant.

Blunt and penetrating injuries constitute only 10% of all oesophageal perforations. In general, the diagnosis may be harder to confirm as pneumomediastinum may be limited to a few small bubbles of air, often with a small associated effusion. Perforation may be confirmed with a water-soluble contrast swallow examination.

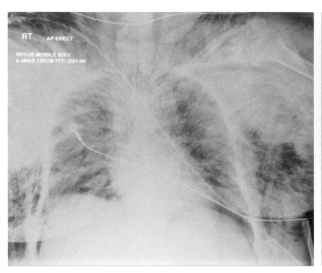

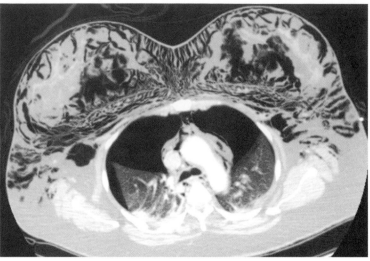

(a)   (b)

Figure 3.17 Iatrogenic tracheal injury following traumatic intubation. (a) Extensive pneumomediastinum and surgical emphysema is present associated with hyperlucency over both diaphragms; (b) CT scan confirms bilateral pneumothoraces, pneumomediastinum and surgical emphysema.

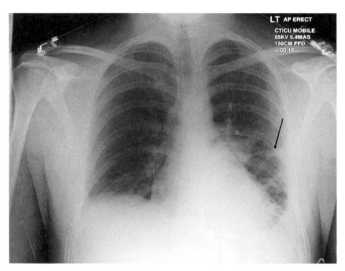

Figure 3.18 Left diaphragmatic rupture with herniation of the splenic flexure (arrow) into the left hemithorax.

Diaphragmatic injury

Diaphragmatic tears due to blunt trauma are thought to occur during compressive abdominal injury resulting in raised intra-abdominal pressure. The incidence is higher on the left side, particularly laterally, as the liver provides support to the right hemidiaphragm. On chest radiography helpful diagnostic features include associated herniation of bowel into the pleural space, or the tip of a nasogastric tube projected over the thorax (Figure 3.18). Non-specific presentations such as elevation of the diaphragm with associated pleural fluid or atelectasis are common. As there is a significant late presentation of these patients with late bowel incarceration, early investigation by CT is advised.

CT is performed with thin section data acquisition with coronal and sagittal reformations. The diaphragmatic injury may be appar-

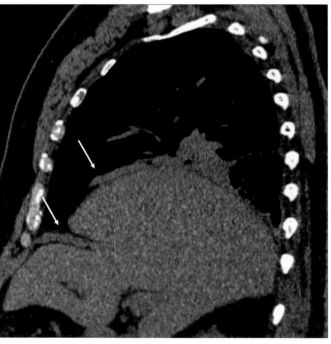

Figure 3.19 Right diaphragmatic injury evaluation by sagittal CT reconstruction demonstrates thickening and retraction of the residual diaphragmatic surface leaves (arrows) and herniation of the liver through the defect.

ent as an area of lack of integrity of the diaphragm, focal diaphragmatic thickening or herniation of abdominal contents (Figure 3.19) The narrowed appearance of the herniated contents at the point of disruption is termed the "collar" or "waist" sign. Herniated contents usually lie posteriorly, resulting in an appearance termed the "dependent viscera" sign, due to the lack of interposition of lung or pleura between the herniated contents and the chest wall (Figure 3.20).

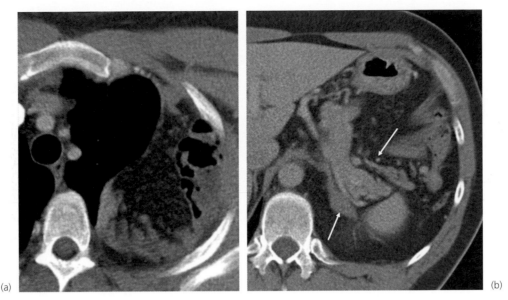

(a)   (b)

Figure 3.20 (a) Left diaphragmatic hernia demonstrates apposition of the herniated contents to the chest wall – "dependent viscera sign"; (b) more inferiorly the herniated contents pass through a narrow "waist" or "collar" formed by the thickened residual diaphragm (arrows).

Penetrating injury to the diaphragm may be very difficult to establish, particularly on the right side, where herniation is less common as the liver abuts the defect. In these instances CT has reduced sensitivity, and any area of focal thickening and associated local haemorrhage should be considered as suspicious, requiring further evaluation by exploratory surgery or further evaluation by magnetic resonance imaging (MRI). Indeed any penetrating injury between the nipple and the naval should be considered to be in both cavities until excluded.

Further reading

Mirvis SE. Diagnostic imaging of acute thoracic injury. *Seminars in Ultrasound, CT, and MRI* 2004; **25**: 156–179.

Sammer M, Wang E, Blackmore CC, Burdick TR & Hollingworth W. Indeterminate CT angiography in blunt thoracic trauma: is CT angiography enough? *American Journal of Roentgenology* 2007; **189**: 603–608.

Shanmuganathan K & Matsumoto J. Imaging of penetrating chest trauma. *Radiologic Clinics of North America* 2006; **44**: 225–238.

Westra SJ & Wallace EC. Imaging evaluation of pediatric chest trauma. *Radiologic Clinics of North America* 2005; **43**: 267–281.

CHAPTER 4

Abdominal Trauma

Niall Power[1] and Mark W. Bowyer[2]

[1]St Bartholomew's and The Royal London Hospitals, London, UK
[2]Uniformed Services University of the Health Sciences, Bethesda, MD, USA

OVERVIEW

- Multidetector computed tomography is the mainstay of imaging the abdomen in the trauma patient. Intravenous contrast-enhanced images in the portal venous phase are usually sufficient, although delayed scans post contrast may occasionally be required. Oral contrast is rarely necessary.

- Solid organ injury may manifest on computed tomography as intraparenchymal or subcapsular haematoma, laceration or infarction. Contained vascular injury or active extravasation may be indicators for angiography and embolization

- Lacerations to the liver carry the risk of injury to central vessels or the biliary tree, in which case a biloma can develop; renal lacerations may cause a urinoma to form if the collecting system is injured

- Gastrointestinal tract injuries can be subtle and are suggested by focal wall thickening. Signs of full thickness injury include free air, but are rarely seen

- Injury to the pancreas is clinically very significant if the pancreatic duct is lacerated or transected

- Diaphragmatic injury can present either acutely or in a delayed manner and multiplanar reformats are useful to make this diagnosis

---

Abdominal trauma may be blunt or penetrating. Blunt trauma is more common in the UK and usually due to road traffic accidents or falls, with resulting compression and deceleration injuries often associated with injuries to the head, spine and limbs. In this situation, abdominal injuries can be missed, with up to 70% of patients having either neurological impairment or a distracting injury, and clinical findings can be misleading in up to 50% of patients. Although less common, penetrating trauma is on the increase, particularly in urban areas.

Simultaneous therapeutic and diagnostic measures need to be instituted on arrival in the resuscitation room. Plain abdominal radiographs have no role in assessment of blunt abdominal trauma but may be useful in penetrating injury to demonstrate bullets or fragments (Figure 4.1). Focused abdominal of sonography in

trauma (FAST) scanning can be performed rapidly and concurrently with other procedures in the resuscitation room to look for free intraperitoneal or intrathoracic fluid, and can triage a haemodynamically unstable patient to surgery. However, it is insufficiently sensitive to exclude solid organ, mesenteric or retroperitoneal injury.

The mainstay of imaging following abdominal trauma is multidetector computed tomography (MDCT). All haemodynamically stable patients with evidence of abdominal trauma (including a positive FAST scan), and all adult polytrauma patients in whom the abdomen cannot be satisfactorily cleared clinically, should have CT. MDCT has a high accuracy (over 95%) for significant abdominopelvic injury and is one of the major factors responsible for the increased use of non-operative management in trauma patients.

Multidetector computed tomography protocols

Trauma CT protocols vary slightly between institutions; however, abdominal images are usually obtained around 60–65 s after an intravenous bolus injection of iodinated contrast (e.g. 100 ml of 300 mg/ml at 3 ml per second). The 60–65 s delay represents the portal venous phase of imaging and gives an optimal trade-off between vascular opacification and solid organ enhancement. The CT raw data are reconstructed on a soft tissue algorithm at both 1.5 mm and 5 mm sections, and in addition multiplanar reformats (MPRs) are routinely reconstructed at 5 mm sections in the coronal plane. MPRs are very useful in trauma assessment for an overview and for depiction of anatomical disruption in the cephalocaudal plane, for example diaphragmatic rupture. Bony algorithm reconstructions of the axial images should also be obtained and may be used to provide coronal and sagittal MPRs of the spine and pelvis. Further reconstructions, such as thin-section sagittal or coronal MPRs, maximum intensity projection scans (MIPs) which are useful particularly for CT angiography and 3D reformats such as volume-rendered images, can be subsequently generated at the discretion of the reporting radiologist.

Unenhanced CT images are rarely required, although they may have to be obtained if there is a contraindication to intravenous contrast with a resulting reduction in sensitivity for organ injury. Delayed scans 5–10 min after contrast injection, while not per-

---

ABC of Imaging in Trauma. By Leonard J. King and David C. Wherry
Published 2010 by Blackwell Publishing

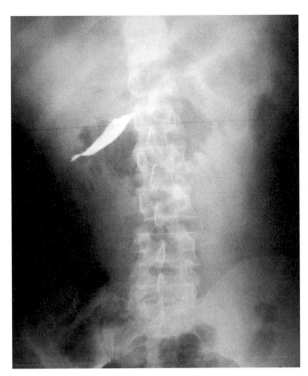

Figure 4.1 Plain abdominal radiograph demonstrating an intra-abdominal metal fragment from an improvised explosive device.

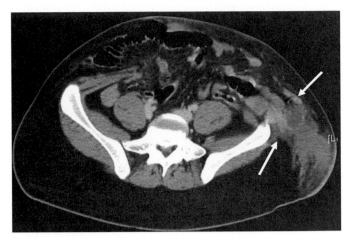

Figure 4.2 CT scan demonstrating on left inferior lumbar hernia in a male patient with blunt abdominal trauma (arrow) following a motor vehicle collision. A midline abdominal wall hernia is also present.

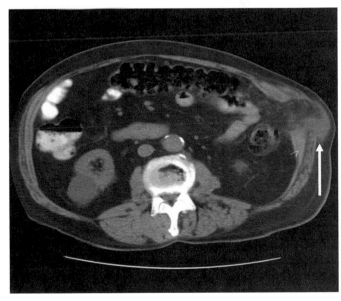

Figure 4.3 Elderly male with blunt trauma following a fall on to his walking stick. CT scan demonstrates a full thickness tear of the abdominal wall muscles with omental fat herniation and a small amount of associated haematoma (arrow).

formed routinely, can be useful to differentiate active bleeding from contained vascular injury and to assess the integrity of the urinary tract, which should be opacified with contrast on delayed images.

Oral contrast is no longer routinely used in most institutions and rectal contrast is usually only used if there is specific concern about colonic trauma either on an initial CT scan or based on the mechanism of injury.

Abdominal wall trauma

The key role of CT in penetrating trauma is to determine whether the peritoneum has been breached, with the associated increased risk of bowel or mesenteric injury. Stranding of the fat planes deep to the site of injury is suggestive of possible peritoneal injury. However, trauma to the abdominal wall itself can be associated with significant haematoma formation, particularly if an abdominal wall vessel such as the inferior epigastric artery is injured.

Abdominal wall disruption from blunt trauma is rare, but important to recognise due to the high frequency of associated intra-abdominal injuries, particularly of the bowel and mesentery. Rapid deceleration in a vehicle collision can cause the lap portion of a seat belt to slip above the pelvis with the deceleration force imparted on to the abdominal wall muscles. This force, in association with pelvic rotation and resulting shearing forces, can cause the development of an acute wall tear with hernia formation. The commonest sites of herniation are posteriorly, in the superior or inferior lumbar triangles (Figure 4.2). The superior lumbar triangle is bordered by the 12th rib superiorly, the internal oblique muscle

anteriorly and the erector spinae muscle posteriorly. The inferior lumbar triangle is bordered by the iliac crest inferiorly, the external oblique muscle anteriorly and the latissimus dorsi muscle posteriorly. Fat and bowel can herniate through abdominal wall defects with the risk of obstruction and strangulation. Occasionally, a direct blow to the abdomen can cause a focal tear in the abdominal wall musculature (Figure 4.3).

Spleen

The spleen is the most commonly injured solid organ following abdominal trauma. Recognition of its vital role in immune function plus increased complications and longer hospital stays

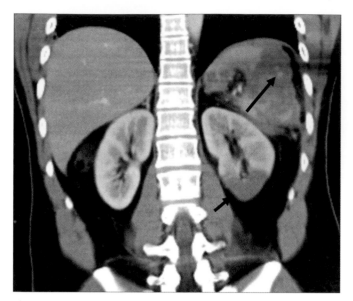

Figure 4.4 Coronal CT scan MPR demonstrating an intraparenchymal splenic haematoma with several focal areas of increased attenuation consistent with bleeding points (long arrow). Perisplenic haematoma is also present and there is traumatic devascularization of the lower pole of the left kidney (short arrow).

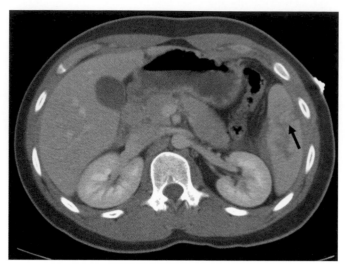

Figure 4.5 CT scan demonstrating splenic lacerations with an associated perisplenic haematoma. The more anterior laceration contains an area of active contrast extravasation (arrow).

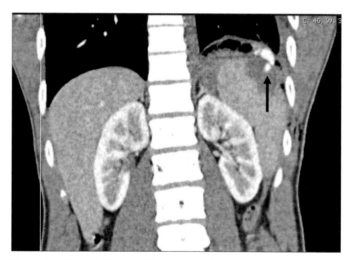

Figure 4.6 Coronal CT scan MPR demonstrating an intraparenchymal splenic haematoma with active contrast extravasation (arrow). Diaphragmatic rupture is evident by the acute bleeding into the left pleural space.

following splenectomy have led to an increased drive for non-operative management of splenic trauma, which is dependent on accurate CT diagnosis and, where necessary, embolization.

Several types of splenic injury can occur: intraparenchymal and subcapsular haematoma, laceration, active extravasation, contained vascular injury and infarction. Clotted blood has an attenuation of approximately 45–70 Hounsfield units (HU), while unclotted blood has an attenuation of 30–45 HU. Acute intraparenchymal haematoma manifests on contrast-enhanced CT as a poorly defined, rounded low attenuation area relative to background splenic parenchyma (Figure 4.4). Subcapsular haematoma is also relatively hypodense with an elliptical shape, conforming to the contour of the spleen and compressing underlying splenic parenchyma. This latter feature is useful to differentiate it from perisplenic haematoma.

A splenic laceration appears as a linear or branching low-density defect on CT (Figure 4.5). Multiple lacerations can give rise to the appearance of a shattered spleen, while a laceration with perisplenic or free intraperitoneal blood implies a capsular tear. Active arterial extravasation or bleeding manifests as an irregular area of increased density relative to background spleen. Typically the attenuation value is within 10 HU of the adjacent artery. Active extravasation can occur into splenic parenchyma, or into a subcapsular or perisplenic haematoma (Figure 4.6).

Contained vascular injury may be either an arteriovenous fistula or a pseudoaneurysm. In the latter there is a tear in the artery, but bleeding is typically limited by the arterial adventitia. On single-phase scanning it can be difficult to differentiate active extravasation from contained vascular injury; however, on 5-minute delayed scans, an area of active extravasation will remain hyperdense and enlarge, whereas a contained vascular injury will typically "wash

out" and be isodense or slightly hypodense relative to splenic parenchyma.

Both active bleeding and contained vascular injury may well be indications for splenic angiography and embolization, in the case of the former to minimize blood loss and in the case of the latter to minimize the risk of delayed rupture with further bleeding.

Splenic infarcts are typically due to an arterial intimal tear with resulting thrombosis giving rise to a peripheral, well-defined, wedge-shaped area of reduced enhancement on CT with its base against the capsular surface (Figure 4.7). They usually heal spontaneously with no sequelae.

Delayed splenic rupture is a rare complication of trauma to the spleen, with relatively high reported mortality rates of up to 15% of cases. Patients usually present around 48 hours or more after the

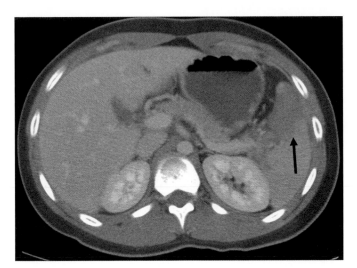

Figure 4.7 CT scan demonstrating a wedge-shaped area of low attenuation within the spleen (arrow) with the base against the capsular surface consistent with a splenic infarct.

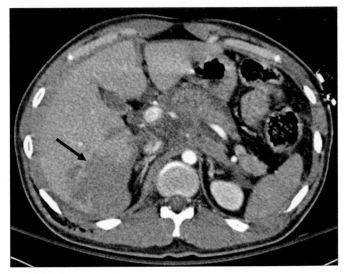

Figure 4.8 Axial CT image demonstrating an intraparenchymal liver haematoma in segment 6 (arrow). No active bleeding is seen though there is some perihepatic haematoma and further haematoma around the pancreatic head.

Box 4.1 **American Association for the Surgery of Trauma (AAST) organ injury severity scale grading system for splenic injury**

Grade 1 Small subcapsular haematoma, less than 10% of surface area

Grade 2 Moderate subcapsular haematoma on 10–50% of surface area; intraparenchymal haematoma less than 5 cm in diameter; capsular laceration less than 1 cm deep

Grade 3 Large or expanding subcapsular haematoma on greater than 50% of surface area; intraparenchymal haematoma greater than 5 cm diameter; capsular laceration 1–3 cm deep

Grade 4 Laceration greater than 3 cm deep; laceration involving segmental or hilar vessels producing major devascularization (>25%)

Grade 5 Shattered spleen; hilar injury that devascularizes the spleen

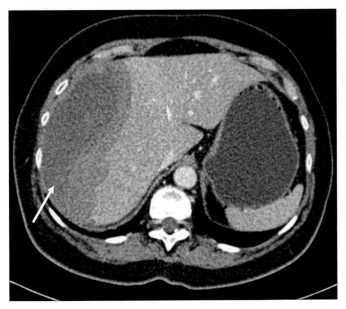

Figure 4.9 Axial CT image demonstrating a heterogenous, subcapsular haematoma (arrow) which is compressing the liver with retention of the normal liver contour. The blood around the periphery is of slightly higher density and is probably clotted.

initial trauma with abdominal symptoms and signs of intraperitoneal haemorrhage due to rupture of a slowly expanding subcapsular haematoma or secondary haemorrhage following dislodgement of a perisplenic haematoma.

While severity of splenic injury according to the American Association for the Surgery of Trauma (AAST) (Box 4.1) does correlate with outcome, this classification does not take account of active extravasation or contained vascular injury such as arteriovenous fistula or pseudoaneurysm formation, and several authors have devised alternative CT-based grading systems, though none has yet been widely adopted.

Liver

The liver is the second most commonly injured organ in abdominal trauma. Between 70 and 90% of hepatic injuries are minor, with the right lobe most commonly affected. The liver is prone to the same array of injuries as the spleen, including intraparenchymal (Figure 4.8) and subcapsular haematoma (Figure 4.9), lacerations (Figure 4.10), infarcts, active extravasation and contained vascular injury.

The AAST liver trauma grading system (Box 4.2) correlates with outcome, but as with the spleen does not take account of active

extravasation (Figure 4.11) or contained vascular injury. Most liver injuries heal spontaneously within 3 months, however, and non-operative management is usually successful.

While liver and splenic injuries share certain characteristics on CT, there are several key issues in imaging hepatic trauma that must be borne in mind. The location of liver lacerations is vital to patient outcome. Lacerations near the major hepatic veins or inferior vena cava (IVC) can be associated with injury to these vessels resulting in catastrophic bleeding with resultant high mortality, particularly if the liver is mobilized at laparotomy. If a laceration occurs in the "bare area" of the liver, posteriorly in the right lobe, haemorrhage can occur into the retroperitoneum, which is

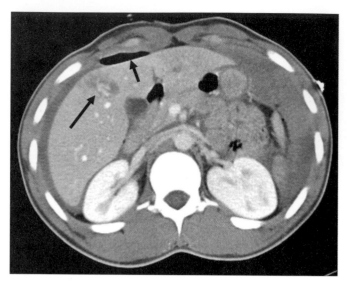

Figure 4.10 Axial CT image demonstrating a laceration within segment 4b of the liver with a central area of active extravasation (long arrow). Both haemoperitoneum and pneumoperitoneum due to a small bowel perforation (short arrow) are also present.

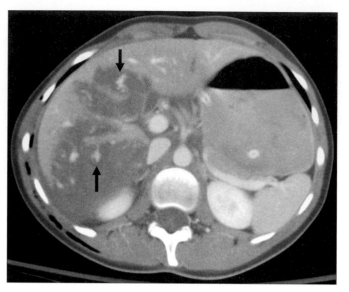

Figure 4.11 CT scan demonstrating several large intraparenchymal haematomas with multiple foci of active contrast extravasation (arrows).

Box 4.2 American Association for the Surgery of Trauma (AAST) organ injury severity scale grading system for liver injury

Grade I	Haematoma	Subcapsular, <10% surface area
	Laceration	Capsular tear <1 cm parenchymal depth
Grade 2	Haematoma	Subcapsular, 10–50% surface area; Intraparenchymal, <10 cm diameter
	Laceration	1–3 cm parenchymal depth, <10 cm in length
Grade 3	Haematoma	Subcapsular, >50% surface area or expanding; ruptured subcapsular or parenchymal haematoma Intraparenchymal haematoma > 10 cm or expanding
	Laceration	>3 cm parenchymal depth
Grade 4	Laceration	Parenchymal disruption involving 25–75% of hepatic lobe or 1–3 Couinaud's segments within a single lobe
Grade 5	Laceration	Parenchymal disruption involving >75% of hepatic lobe or >3 Couinaud's segments within a single lobe
	Vascular	Juxtahepatic venous injuries; i.e., retrohepatic vena cava/central major hepatic veins
Grade 6	Vascular	Hepatic avulsion

NB: Advance one grade for multiple injuries, up to grade 3

frequently associated with injury to the right adrenal and kidney. A FAST scan may be falsely negative in this setting. Lacerations involving the porta hepatis may be associated with a tear in the central biliary tree, which can lead to the development of a biloma, which manifests as an enlarging perihepatic fluid collection on subsequent CT. This may necessitate percutaneous drainage or covered stent placement in the common bile duct. Ongoing bile leak can be diagnosed either by aspirating the fluid or with a nuclear medicine hepatobiliary imino-diacetic acid (HIDA) scan (Figure 4.12). Biliary peritonitis can also occur and is manifest on

CT as thickened enhancing peritoneum with free fluid, in the presence of a bile leak. The other main delayed complication following liver trauma is development of an intrahepatic abscess, which is more common following surgery or embolization and can generally be drained percutaneously. Delayed liver rupture is very rare.

Genitourinary tract

The kidney is the most commonly injured urologic organ following trauma, although 80% of injuries are minor and heal spontaneously. The kidney is prone to the same range of solid organ injuries as the spleen and liver, namely contusions, subcapsular and perinephric haematoma, lacerations, active extravasation, contained vascular injury and infarcts, which have the same radiological appearances as previously described. As for the liver and spleen, the AAST grading system (Box 4.3) does not take active extravasation and contained vascular injury into account.

A useful clinical indicator is the presence of haematuria, which is present in 95% of significant renal injuries, but can be absent in renal vascular injuries, or injury to the pelviureteric junction (PUJ) or ureter. Contusions are common, accounting for 80% of injuries. Subcapsular haematomas are rare, due to the strong attachment of the renal capsule, but if large can compress the kidney sufficiently to cause excessive renin secretion and hypertension – the "Page kidney". Perinephric haematomas lie between the kidney and Gerota's fascia and are commoner than subcapsular haematomas. Lacerations are linear or branching low-density areas (Figure 4.13) and if they reach the hilum of the kidney delayed scanning is indicated to look for a urine leak (Figure 4.14). Urinoma can be treated via percutaneous drainage or with a ureteric stent. Most renal injuries are treated conservatively, with angiography and embolization reserved for active extravasation or contained vascular injury, ideally to conserve as much functioning renal tissue as possible. Main or segmental renal artery injury can occur due to thrombosis secondary to an intimal tear, dissection or arterial laceration and can cause devascularization of the entire kidney, or segmental infarcts (Figure 4.4), which usually resolve spontaneously.

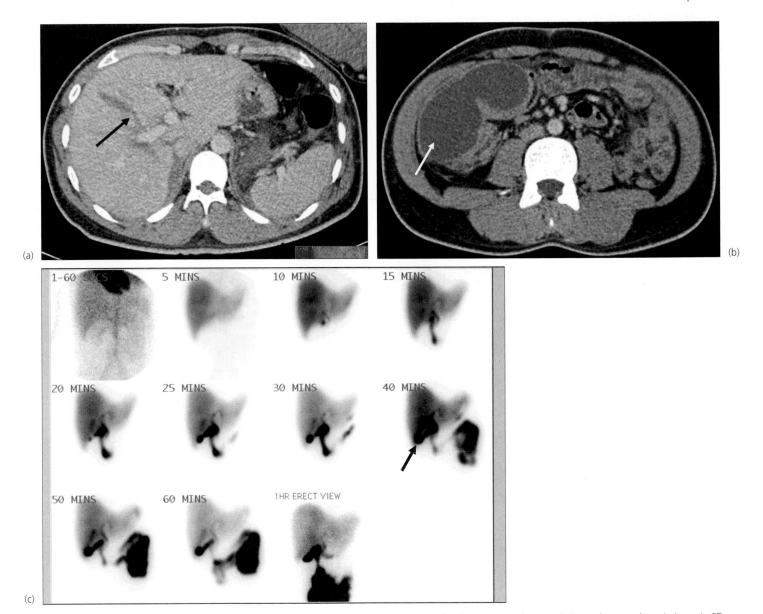

Figure 4.12 Evolution of a traumatic biloma. The initial CT scan (a) demonstrates a central liver laceration in close proximity to the porta hepatis (arrow). CT one month later (b) demonstrates a low-attenuation fluid collection in the right flank (arrow). A subsequent HIDA scan (c) shows leakage of bile from the biliary tree into the collection (arrow), which was drained percutaneously.

Box 4.3 **American Association for the Surgery of Trauma (AAST) organ injury severity scale grading system for kidney injury**

Grade 1   Contusion or contained and non-expanding subcapsular haematoma, without parenchymal laceration; haematuria

Grade 2   Non-expanding, confined, perirenal haematoma or cortical laceration less than 1 cm deep; no urinary extravasation

Grade 3   Parenchymal laceration extending more than 1 cm into cortex; no collecting system rupture or urinary extravasation

Grade 4   Parenchymal laceration extending through the renal cortex, medulla and collecting system

Grade 5   Pedicle injury or avulsion of renal hilum that devascularizes the kidney; completely shattered kidney; thrombosis of the main renal artery

Ureteric injury is rare and typically occurs at the PUJ. It can either be a complete or partial tear; if contrast is seen in the distal ureter on delayed scans this implies an incomplete tear. Stenting is indicated if a large tear occurs.

Bladder injury may be limited to wall contusion or haematoma, but bladder rupture can occur, which may be either intra- or extra-peritoneal. Bladder rupture can be diagnosed with either conventional cystography or CT cystography, where dilute contrast is instilled into the bladder via a Foley catheter. Intraperitoneal rupture usually occurs due to a direct blow to a distended bladder and necessitates surgical repair as the patient is at risk of peritonitis. Extraperitoneal rupture (Figure 4.15) is usually due to laceration of the bladder wall from pelvic fracture fragments and can be treated conservatively with catheter placement.

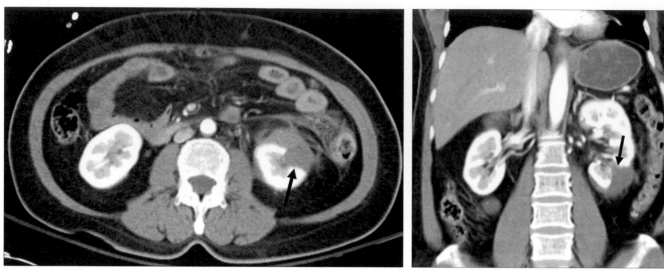

(a)

(b)

Figure 4.13 Axial (a) and coronal MPR (b) CT images demonstrating a left lower pole renal laceration (arrows) with an associated perinephric haematoma.

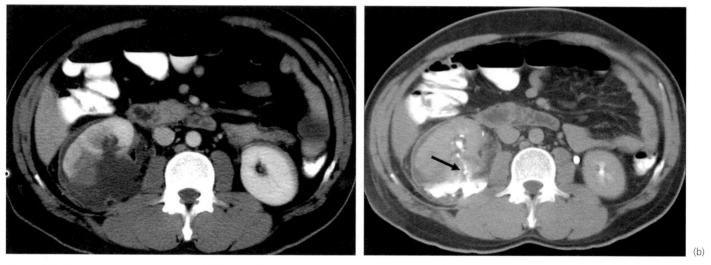

(a)

(b)

Figure 4.14 Venous phase contrast-enhanced CT image (a) demonstrates a large laceration that reaches the right renal hilum with associated perinephric fluid. Delayed axial CT image 10 minutes post contrast (b) demonstrates leakage of contrast opacified urine into the perinephric fluid collection (arrow) confirming the presence of a traumatic urinoma. Absence of contrast in the right ureter is also demonstrated.

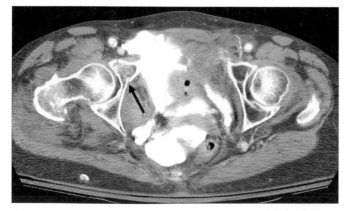

Figure 4.15 Axial CT image following instillation of dilute contrast into the bladder via a Foley catheter demonstrates extensive leakage of contrast into the perivesical spaces consistant with extraperitoneal bladder rupture. A fracture of the anterior column of the right acetabulum (arrow) is also present.

Adrenal trauma is commoner on the right and is usually associated with other injuries. CT signs include a haematoma expanding or obliterating the normal gland contour (Figure 4.16), or active extravasation. Unilateral adrenal trauma rarely causes long-term problems, but bilateral trauma can cause long-term adrenal insufficiency.

Gastrointestinal tract

Free intra-abdominal fluid in the absence of solid organ injury is suggestive of injury to the bowel or mesentery, particularly in a male patient or a female patient with large amounts of free fluid, or fluid between the leaves of the mesentery. The commonest sites for free fluid to accumulate are Morrison's pouch, the perisplenic region, the paracolic gutters and the pouch of Douglas.

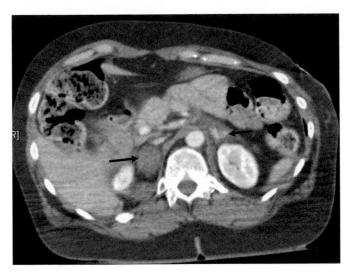

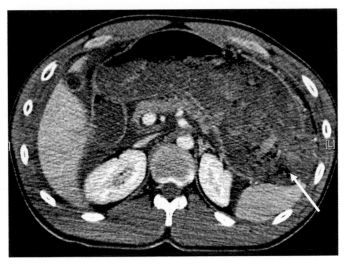

Figure 4.16 Axial CT image of the upper abdomen demonstrating bilateral adrenal haemorrhages (arrows) following blunt abdominal trauma.

Figure 4.17 Axial CT image through the stomach demonstrating a full-thickness tear of the gastric fundus with some spilling of gastric contents into the peritoneal cavity (arrow).

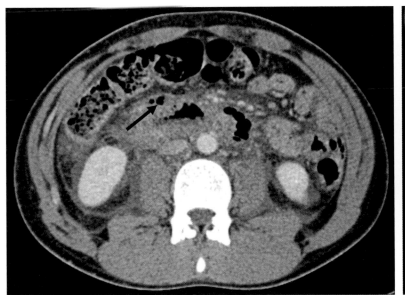

(a)

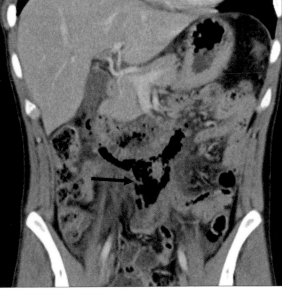

(b)

Figure 4.18 Traumatic duodenal laceration. Axial (a) and coronal MPR (b) CT images demonstrate free retroperitoneal air (arrows) extending into the root of the small bowel mesentery and thickening of the adjacent duodenum. A tear in the third part of the duodenum was confirmed at laparotomy.

Gastric trauma

Blunt trauma to the stomach is relatively rare, and most commonly involves the fundus. It is usually due to high-velocity impact on a full stomach. As in other parts of the gastrointestinal tract, injuries can be full or partial thickness. Full-thickness injury can lead to gastric rupture with pneumoperitoneum (Figure 4.17). Partial-thickness injury can be either serosal or mucosal; the latter can cause haematemesis. Luminal air can also dissect into gastric veins causing portal pneumatosis, which may give the misleading impression of bowel wall infarction. The stomach abuts the left hemidiaphragm and thus gastric trauma may be associated with

diaphragmatic rupture, which can predispose to intrathoracic gastric migration with possible volvulus and strangulation.

Bowel injury

The small bowel is most commonly injured, particularly where it is relatively fixed at the ligament of Treitz and distal ileum, resulting in a wall contusion, serosal tear or full-thickness tear. Wall contusion or serosal tear may manifest as a focal area of bowel wall thickening, which may be eccentric or concentric. Full-thickness tears can give rise to pneumoperitoneum or retroperitoneal free air (Figure 4.18), intramural air, wall discontinuity and extraluminal oral contrast (if used) or bowel content (Figure 4.19). Delayed diagnosis may give rise to peritonitis. Focal small bowel wall thickening must be distinguished from the diffuse small bowel wall thickening sometimes seen as part of the hypovolaemic shock complex, other signs of which include small bowel mucosal hyperenhancement due to increased vascular permeability (Figure 4.20), peripancreatic fluid, hyperenhancing adrenal glands and flattening of the IVC.

Mesenteric injury may manifest on CT as mesenteric fat stranding or haematoma, active extravasation into the mesentery (Figure 4.21) or signs of mesenteric vascular injury, including abrupt vessel termination and vascular beading. The latter can lead to bowel ischemia and infarction, while a mesenteric tear can give rise to a subsequent internal hernia.

Pancreas

Trauma to the pancreas is rare but can lead to significant complications such as abscess or pseudocyst formation, pancreatitis or pancreatic fistula. The key issue in pancreatic trauma is the integrity of the pancreatic duct. Signs of pancreatic injury can be subtle on CT, which most commonly demonstrates peripancreatic fluid and

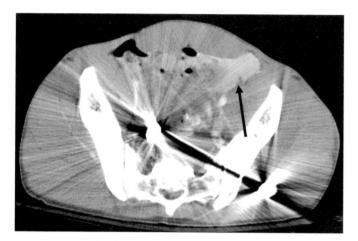

Figure 4.19 Rectal perforation following a gunshot wound to the pelvis. Axial CT image with intravenous and rectal contrast demonstrates extensive leakage of rectal contrast (arrow). Metallic artefact from the bullet fragments is also demonstrated.

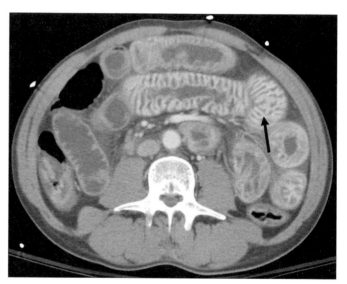

Figure 4.20 Contrast-enhanced axial CT image demonstrating prominent small bowel wall thickening and mucosal hyperenhancement due to increased vascular permeability (arrow) as result of hypovolaemic shock. Free intraperitoneal fluid is also present.

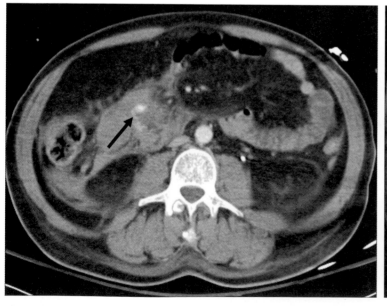

(a)

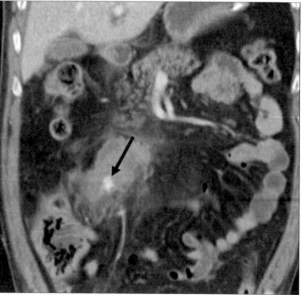

(b)

Figure 4.21 Axial (a) and coronal MPR (b) CT images demonstrating a mesenteric haematoma with a central focus of active contrast extravasation (arrows).

fat stranding, although peripancreatic changes can also be due to fluid resuscitation. Contusion to the gland may cause diffuse swelling, while a laceration is manifest as a linear low-attenuation defect. If a laceration involves more than 50% of the anteroposterior diameter of the gland there is an increased risk of ductal injury (Figure 4.22). Complete pancreatic transection may occur but this can be difficult to detect unless there is fluid or blood between the transected edges. Duct rupture can be diagnosed non-invasively with magnetic resonance cholangiopancreatography (MRCP), which also allows visualization of the ducts upstream from a disruption; endoscopic retrograde cholangiopancreatography (ERCP), however, offers the opportunity both for diagnosis and treatment via covered stent placement.

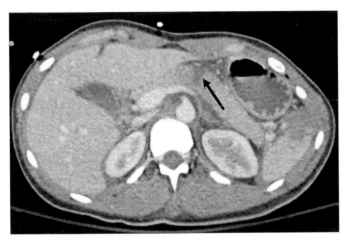

Figure 4.22 Contrast-enhanced axial CT image demonstrating a vertical laceration at the junction of the neck and body of the pancreas (arrow). The laceration extends over approximately 75% of the anteroposterior diameter of the gland and is likely to be associated with pancreatic duct injury. An intraparenchymal splenic haematoma is also present.

Gallbladder and extrahepatic bile duct

Gallbladder injuries are rare, due to the protective effect of the overlying liver, and may be difficult to diagnose. There is an increased risk of injury if the gallbladder is distended at the time of trauma. Gallbladder injuries include contusion, laceration, perforation and avulsion. CT signs include pericholecystic fluid, which as with peripancreatic fluid may be non-specific, gallbladder wall thickening and loss of clarity, a gallbladder wall tear and active extravasation into the lumen. In avulsion, the gallbladder is displaced from its normal fossa and can lie anywhere in the peritoneal cavity. The treatment of choice for significant gallbladder injury is cholecystectomy.

Extrahepatic bile duct injury from blunt trauma is rare but may occur at sites of anatomic fixation such as within the pancreatic head. Acute deceleration with compression of the duct against the spine can cause ductal transection, and elevation of the liver in blunt trauma can cause stretching of the duct. As in intrahepatic bile duct injury, biloma may ensue, manifesting as a perihepatic fluid collection on CT. Treatment may be either with open surgical repair or stent placement at ERCP.

Diaphragm

Diaphragmatic rupture is rare and commoner on the left. It can be subtle at the time of initial imaging and MPRs are very useful in diagnosis. Several signs of diaphragmatic rupture have been described, including focal diaphragmatic discontinuity and thickening, loss of diaphragmatic clarity, visceral herniation into the chest, the "collar" sign (Figure 4.23) where there is narrowing of a viscus, usually the stomach as it traverses the diaphragmatic defect, and the dependent viscera sign, where a tear causes the solid organs of the upper abdomen to lie against the posterior chest wall in the supine position. While rare, diagnosis is important as delayed presentation with gastric or colonic obstruction or strangulation can have up to 60% mortality.

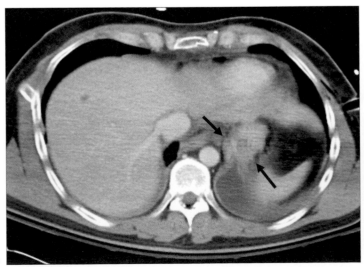

(a)

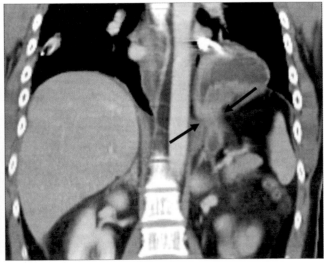

(b)

Figure 4.23 Diaphragmatic rupture. Axial (a) and coronal MPR (b) CT images demonstrating the "collar sign" of a diaphragmatic tear with narrowing of the stomach as it traverses the diaphragmatic defect (arrows).

Further reading

Brofman N, Atri M, Hanson JM, Grinblat L, Chughtai T & Brenneman F. Evaluation of bowel and mesenteric trauma with multidetector CT. *Radiographics* 2006; **26**: 1119–1131.

Miller LA & Shanmuganathan K. Multidetector CT evaluation of abdominal trauma. *Radiologic Clinics of North America* 2005; **43**: 1079–1095.

Shanmuganathan K. Multi-detector row CT imaging of blunt abdominal trauma. *Seminars in Ultrasound CT and MRI* 2004; **25**: 180–204.

Stuhlfaut JW, Anderson SW & Soto JA. Blunt abdominal trauma: current imaging techniques and CT findings in patients with solid organ, bowel and mesenteric injury. *Seminars in Ultrasound CT and MRI* 2007; **28**: 115–129.

Yoon W, Jeong YY, Kim JK, Seo JJ, Lim HS, Shin SS *et al*. CT in blunt liver trauma. *Radiographics* 2005; **25**: 87–104.

CHAPTER 5

Pelvic Trauma

Madeleine Sampson and Gavin Bowyer

Southampton University Hospitals NHS Trust, Southampton, Hampshire, UK

OVERVIEW

- Pelvic injury involves bony and ligament disruption and is a marker of serious trauma, frequently associated with injury to the head, spine and intra-abdominal organs

- Features on the plain anteroposterior radiograph of the pelvis allow accurate assessment of direction of force and severity of trauma

- Classification of pelvic fractures depends on stability and direction of force, and knowledge of these factors predicts injury patterns, resuscitation requirements and prognosis

- Unstable injuries (involving at least two areas of the pelvic ring, either bone or soft tissue) should be investigated with computed tomography

- Haemorrhage is the most serious early life-threatening complication. If arterial, it may be amenable to transcatheter embolisation and, more commonly, if venous, may be reduced by use of an external binder

---

Box 5.1 Additional injuries associated with pelvic disruption

Closed head injury – 51%
Long bone fracture – 48%
Peripheral nerve injury – 26%
Thoracic injury – 20%
Urethra (male) – 15%
Bladder – 10%
Spleen – 10%
Liver – 7%
GI tract – 7%
Kidney – 7%
Urethra (female) – 6%
Mesentery – 4%
Diaphragm – 2%

Introduction

Injuries to the bony pelvic ring usually occur in high-energy trauma and are often associated with pelvic soft tissue damage and haemorrhage. Pelvic disruption is a marker of serious injury and is strongly associated with major trauma to other body systems, such as head injury, abdominal visceral injury, long bone fractures and spinal injury (Box 5.1). The overall mortality in pelvic ring fractures is between 5 and 10%; however, unstable fractures with associated hypovolaemic shock carry a mortality of greater than 50%. Other serious complications include damage to the urogenital system, neurological injury, hip joint disruption, rectal injury, infection and thrombo-embolic disease. Laparotomy for associated injuries may be required, but is not undertaken lightly as reported series have shown a high complication rate and mortality, even in cases where the laparotomy was negative.

Pelvic fracture classification by direction of force

Pelvic fractures can be classified according to pelvic stability and the mechanism of injury. The modified system described in 1986 by Young, Burgess and Brumback at a major North American trauma centre has proved valuable in predicting injury patterns, resuscitation requirements and prognosis (Table 5.1).

Lateral compression fractures

Between 50 and 70% of pelvic ring fractures occur due to lateral compression and are usually the result of side impact road traffic accidents or crush injuries. These injuries cause an acute reduction in pelvic volume with displacement of fracture fragments towards and sometimes across the midline. The severity of lateral compression fractures varies from Type 1, involving pubic ramus disruption and a buckle fracture of the ipsilateral sacrum (Figure 5.1), through more complex Type 2 ipsilateral injuries, including fractures of the iliac wing or central displacement of the hemipelvis, to Type 3 injuries, which involve central displacement of the ipsilateral pelvis with sacral plus pubic fractures and disruption of the contralateral pelvis which may undergo external rotation producing the so-called "wind swept pelvis" (Figure 5.2). Displacement of sharp bone fragments across the pelvis is associated with a high incidence of soft tissue damage, particularly to the bladder and urethra. Recent quantitative 3D radiographic analysis has

---

ABC of Imaging in Trauma. By Leonard J. King and David C. Wherry
Published 2010 by Blackwell Publishing

Table 5.1 Classification of pelvic fractures by direction of force (based on the Young and Burgess system)

Mechanism and type	Characteristics	Hemipelvis displacement	Stability
AP compression, type I	Pubic diastasis <2.5 cm	External rotation	Stable
AP compression, type II	Pubic diastasis >2.5 cm, anterior sacroiliac joint disruption	External rotation	Rotationally unstable, vertically stable
AP compression, type III	Type II plus posterior sacroiliac joint disruption	External rotation	Rotationally unstable, vertically unstable
Lateral compression, type I	Ipsilateral sacral buckle fracture, ipsilateral horizontal pubic rami fractures (or disruption of symphysis with overlapping pubic bones)	Internal rotation	Stable
Lateral compression, type II	Type I plus ipsilateral iliac wing fracture or posterior sacroiliac joint disruption	Internal rotation	Rotationally unstable, vertically stable
Lateral Compression type III	Force continues across midline to affect the contralateral hemipelvis. Ipsilateral hemipelvis sustains type I or type II injury with associated internal rotation. Contralateral pelvis undergoes external rotation (windswept pelvis)	Ipsilateral internal and contralateral external rotation	Rotationally unstable, vertically stable
Vertical shear	Vertical pubic rami fractures, SI joint disruption +/− adjacent fractures	Vertical (cranial)	Rotationally unstable, vertically unstable

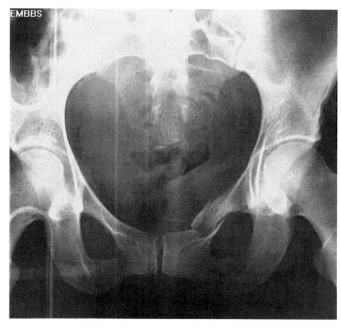

Figure 5.1 Lateral compression Type I Injury with overlapping fractures of the left pubic rami and subtle fractures of the left side of the sacrum visible as a buckling in the outline of the sacral foraminal margins.

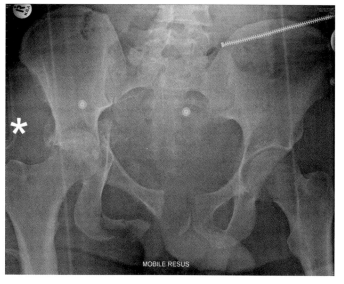

Figure 5.2 Combination injury with pubic rami fractures, disruption of the posterior pelvis and symphysis pubis and rotation of the contralateral pelvis. An associated central acetabular fracture is shown – a well-recognized complication of lateral compression injuries.

contributed to the understanding of lateral compression injuries by demonstrating variations in rotation and translation, which may go some way to explaining the variation in outcomes in this group of fractures.

Anteroposterior (AP) compression fractures

This is the second most common direction of force resulting in pelvic injury. By their very nature these fractures are usually due to compression injuries and can be associated with crush damage to soft tissues. The key features are of widening of the pubic symphysis to greater than 5 mm, and sacroiliac joint disruption. There

is a degree of flexibility in the sacroiliac joints and thus it is possible to widen to pubic symphysis up to 2–2.5 cm before the sacroiliac ligaments are disrupted; it must, however, be borne in mind that the separation at the symphysis shown on imaging may not reflect the magnitude of disruption that was present at the moment of injury. The anterior sacroiliac ligaments give way first and the pelvis opens up producing an "open book injury" (Figure 5.3). The pelvis becomes rotationally unstable if both the anterior and posterior stabilizing joints are disrupted or if the bony ring is fractured at multiple sites. Some of these injury patterns, particularly external rotation, allow the pelvic volume to increase. In addition there is opening up of the pelvic space into the retroperitoneum, perineum and buttocks, producing a large potential space into which bleed-

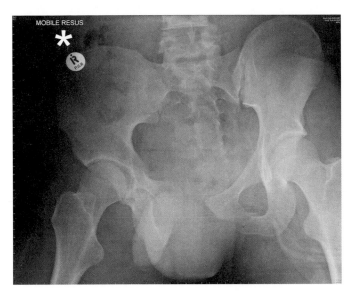

Figure 5.3 Open book injury due to an anterior compression force. The symphysis has opened and there are bilateral pubic rami fractures and disruption of the sacroiliac joints.

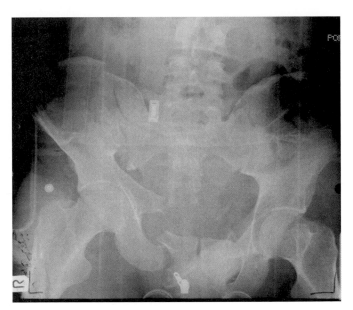

Figure 5.5 Severe bilateral vertical shear fractures with vertical displacement of the hemipelvis and vertically oriented pubic fractures. The posterior fracture on the right passes through the iliac blade.

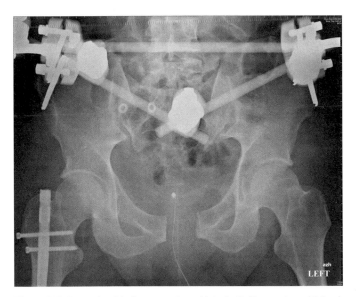

Figure 5.4 External pelvic fixator anchored into both iliac crests and joined anteriorly to stabilize this open book fracture with disrupted sacroiliac joints and symphysis pubis.

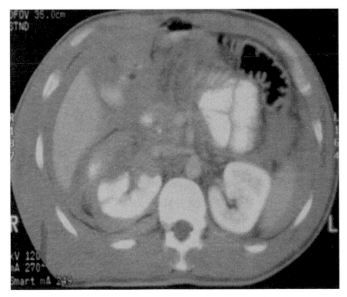

Figure 5.6 Same case as Figure 5.5. The right kidney has been transected by the vertical displacement of the hemipelvis. Note the extensive haemoperitoneum with a large amount of free intraperitoneal fluid.

ing can occur. The disruption of the posterior elements is an indicator of significant trauma to this region, with associated damage to vascular structures, including branches of the iliac arteries and veins. Patients are thus at risk of major pelvic haemorrhage due to the combination of vascular injury, an increased potential volume and reduced ability of the soft tissues to tamponade. Emergency treatment protocols have therefore been developed to reduce the potential volume and stabilize the pelvis using techniques including pelvic binding or external fixation (Figure 5.4).

Vertical shearing fracture

This is the least common direction of force causing pelvic disruptions producing 5 to 15% of pelvic ring injuries. This type of injury is usually due to a fall from a height, landing on the lower limbs (thereby driving one or both halves of the pelvis upwards), or a road traffic accident with head-on collision and lower limb impaction. The key here is that the hemipelvis is displaced in a craniad direction (Figure 5.5). If the injury is complete and the anterior plus posterior ligaments are disrupted it is not unknown for the hemipelvis to travel superiorly as far as the liver on the right and the hemidiaphragm on the left, producing soft tissue shearing, perforation and compression injuries to the abdominal organs. The kidneys are at particular risk of vascular and parenchymal damage (Figure 5.6).

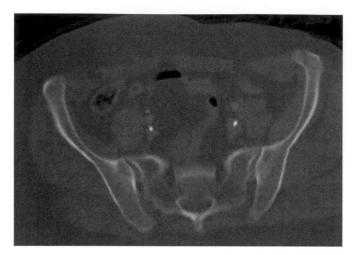

Figure 5.7 Simple iliac wing fracture – the ring structure of the bony pelvis is not disrupted.

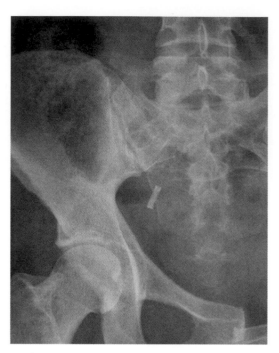

Figure 5.8 Plain radiograph demonstrating a right L5 transverse process in association with a vertical shear fractures of the pelvis involving the right sacral ala.

Pelvic injury stability

In the management of pelvic fractures it is important to recognize the injury pattern and to assess whether the injury is stable to vertical, AP and rotational forces (Table 5.1). There are several additional pelvic fractures that do not involve the bony ring and are therefore not unstable. These include avulsion fractures, iliac wing fractures, isolated sacral fractures and pubic rami fractures, particularly from a direct blow or straddle injury (Figure 5.7).

Imaging of pelvic fractures

AP pelvic radiograph

The supine AP radiograph is the initial imaging investigation for pelvic trauma and is incorporated into the advanced trauma life support (ATLS) primary imaging survey. Inlet and outlet views were previously taken to review the ring configuration of the pelvis but have now been mostly superseded by computed tomography (CT). It is important to note that the plain AP radiograph of the pelvis does not demonstrate the sacrum accurately. Although some sacroiliac disruptions may be evident on the AP film, the degree of subluxation has often reduced by the time the radiograph is obtained.

Careful scrutiny of the AP radiograph allows identification of the main direction and severity of the force underlying the injury, thereby directing the search for associated bony, joint and soft tissue trauma. Vertical displacement of the hemipelvis with vertically oriented pubic rami fractures obviously imply vertical shear force, and the presence of associated soft tissue injuries should be considered. Buckle fracture of the sacrum and horizontally oriented pubic rami fractures suggest a lateral compression force and widening of the pubic symphysis suggests AP compression.

Fractures of the lower lumbar transverse processes may also be demonstrated on pelvic radiographs. While fractures of the transverse processes of L1–L4 are usually regarded as muscular avul-

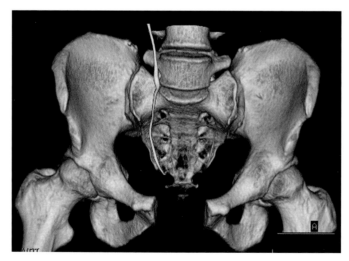

Figure 5.9 3D volume-rendered CT image of an AP compression fracture. The image may be viewed in any orientation.

sions, an avulsion of the transverse process of L5 implies avulsion of the iliolumbar ligaments and associated significant pelvic injury (Figure 5.8).

Computed tomography

CT scanning should now be performed for the assessment of significant pelvic trauma with multiplaner and 3D reformatted images, which can replace inlet, outlet and oblique radiographs (Figure 5.9). CT clearly delineates the posterior pelvis demonstrating sacral fractures and small sacroiliac avulsions accurately. It also allows assessment of pelvic soft tissue injuries and is routinely performed by trauma centres as part of the whole body CT protocol for victims of major trauma.

Other imaging modalities

Magnetic resonance imaging (MRI) is not routinely used to evaluate the acutely fractured pelvis but can be useful for demonstrating radiographically occult fractures and soft tissue avulsions, particularly following sports injuries and low-energy trauma such as falls. Ultrasound also has a limited utility in the investigation of pelvic trauma, although pelvic haematomas are occasionally demonstrated on focused assessment of sonography in trauma (FAST) ultrasound. Ultrasound is also useful in the evaluation of some soft tissue injuries and in the assessment of lower limb deep venous thrombosis. Angiography and endovascular interventional techniques are invaluable and potentially life saving where a pelvic fracture is associated with uncontrolled arterial bleeding.

Complications

Haemorrhage

Haemorrhage is the most serious immediate complication and is most commonly due to venous bleeding from pelvic veins or the marrow spaces at fracture sites. Immediate treatment of haemorrhages to reduce the potential volume is by pelvic binding or fixation.

Pelvic binders have recently increased in popularity as part of the initial management of unstable pelvic fractures. These contribute to tamponade and stabilization of the bony elements. In AP fracture patterns the application of a binder can markedly reduce the symphyseal diastasis. The reduction at the symphysis anteriorly and posteriorly at the sacroiliac joint may give the appearance on CT scanning of a virtually intact pelvic ring; it is important that this is borne in mind when interpreting CT scans or radiographs taken after the application of these devices.

Arterial bleeding, although not the commonest cause of haemorrhage, can be rapidly fatal. This is particularly so when the greater sciatic notch is disrupted with sharp bone fragments and bleeding occurs from branches of the internal iliac artery, most commonly the superior gluteal artery (Figure 5.10). Pelvic transcatheter embolization of disrupted pelvic arteries is less invasive, more successful and associated with fewer complications than an open surgical approach, which by its very nature disrupts physiological tamponade.

Bladder injury

Bladder injury can be a direct complication of a fracture, particularly lateral compression injuries, or an associated injury, as in AP compression trauma, and may occur in the absence of a demonstrable pelvic fracture. Extraperitoneal bladder rupture is the more common injury pattern (Figure 5.11). The less common intraperitoneal rupture is usually due to blunt trauma on a distended bladder. Cystography was previously the imaging method of choice,

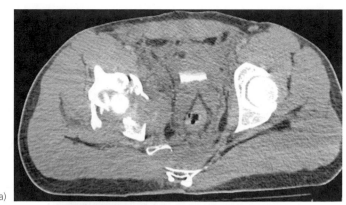

(a)

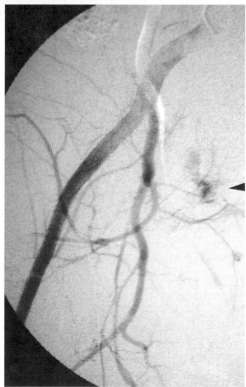

(b)

Figure 5.10 (a) CT image following intravenous contrast showing extravasation of contrast at the site of the comminuted right pelvic fracture; (b) digital subtraction image at the time of subsequent angiography showing the contrast extravasation from the right superior gluteal artery.

but CT with intravenous contrast or CT cystography is now preferred.

Urethral injury

Urethral injury is due to shearing forces, and is much more common in males than females due to the longer length and increased mobility of the urethra. Severity varies from Type 1, where the membranous urethra is stretched and narrowed, through Type 2, where the membranous urethra is disrupted near the neck of the bladder, to Type 3 injuries, where the membranous urethra is extensively disrupted. Involvement of a urologist at an early stage

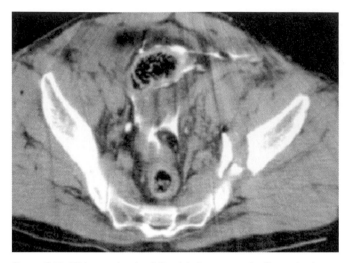

Figure 5.11 CT image showing left pelvic fractures and spillage of urine containing contrast from an earlier intravenous injection following excretion. Note similar density of urine in the ureters.

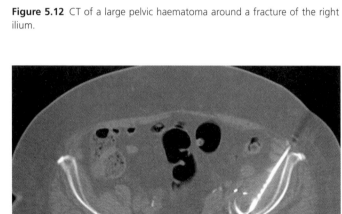

Figure 5.12 CT of a large pelvic haematoma around a fracture of the right ilium.

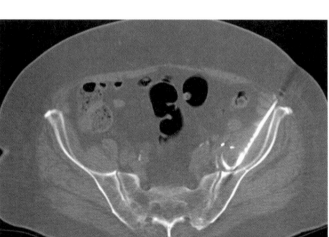

Figure 5.13 CT image of the pelvis demonstrating a pigtail catheter in a left iliacus abscess.

of assessment is important, and retrograde urethrography will aid decision making. While it is possible to by-pass the problem by suprapubic catheterization, this should be regarded as a last resort, as the presence of a suprapubic catheter will severely limit or complicate the surgical approach for anterior pelvic stabilization. Per-urethral catheterization, endoscopically guided if necessary, should be the preferred option.

Neurological injury

Fractures of the posterior pelvis and sacrum can be associated with direct damage to the sacral plexus or sacral roots. Fractures extending into the greater sciatic notch may disrupt the sciatic nerve, and fractures involving the acetabulum may disrupt the sciatic nerve in its extra-pelvic course. These injuries are associated with poorer outcome, through the impairment of lower limb function and may also be associated with significant problems arising from neurogenic pain.

Infection

Pelvic wound infection or infection related to external fixation devices may be problematic. The presence of a pelvic haematoma and possible bacterial soiling from perforation of internal structures can also result in abscess formation. CT scanning is usually the modality of choice for investigation and serial CT scans may be required to assess progress and response to treatment (Figure 5.12) or to guide drainage (Figure 5.13).

Thrombo-embolic disease

The combination of bleeding, possible shock and associated coagulopathy plus immobilization places patients at risk of thrombo-embolic disease. Doppler ultrasonography is the imaging method of choice for investigating deep venous thrombosis in the lower extremities, but assessing pelvic thrombus is difficult and conventional venography or CT may be required.

Acetabular fractures

There are specific fracture patterns relating to the acetabulum, which may occur in isolation or in association with pelvic ring fractures (Table 5.2). The three-dimensional shape of the ball and socket of the hip joint presents difficulties in accurately delineating the pattern of damage on two-dimensional radiography or axial CT images, and multiplanar reformat (MPR) images plus 3D volume-rendered CT image can be very useful. Nonetheless, plain film radiography is still the mainstay of investigation.

The structural components of the acetabulum are the columns, walls, dome and quadrilateral plate. The load-bearing stresses are carried by the anterior and posterior columns. The anterior column is larger, beginning at the iliac wing and extending down the anterior portion of the acetabulum to incorporate the superior pubic ramus. The posterior column begins at the sciatic notch and extends down the posterior acetabulum into the ischium. Both columns are attached to the axial skeleton by the sciatic buttress that connects the acetabulum to the sacroiliac joint. The dome or

Table 5.2 Imaging features of acetabular fractures (Brandser and Marsh, 1988)

Fracture type	Obturator ring fracture	Ilioischial line disrupted	Iliopectineal line disrupted	Iliac wing fracture	Posterior wall fracture	Pelvis into halves	Spur sign	CT fracture orientation
Both columns	Yes	Yes	Yes	Yes	No	Front/back	Yes	Horizontal
Anterior column	Yes	No	Yes	Yes	No	Front/back	No	Horizontal
Posterior column	Yes	Yes	No	No	No	Front/back	No	Horizontal
Posterior column with posterior wall	Yes	Yes	No	No	Yes	Front/back	No	Horizontal
T-shaped	Yes	Yes	Yes	No	No	Top/bottom	No	Vertical
Transverse with posterior wall	No	Yes	Yes	No	Yes	Top/bottom	No	Vertical
Transverse	No	Yes	Yes	No	No	Top/bottom	No	Vertical
Posterior wall	No	No	No	No	Yes	No	No	Oblique
Anterior wall	No	No	Yes	No	No	No	No	Oblique
Anterior column with posterior hemitransverse†	No	Yes	Yes	Yes	No	N/A	No	N/A

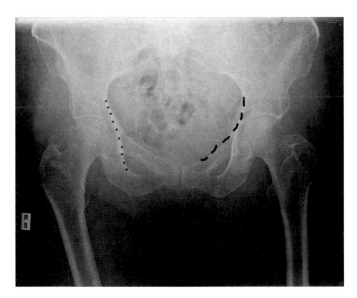

Figure 5.14 Anteroposterior pelvic radiograph demonstrating the iliopectineal line (left side in dashes) and the ilioischial line (right side in dots).

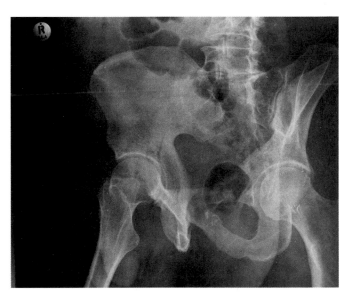

Figure 5.15 Judet oblique view with the left side elevated up (left anterior 45 degree oblique) showing the right posterior column and the left anterior column. This is also known as a right iliac oblique as the iliac wing is well demonstrated.

roof of the acetabulum is the superior aspect, which carries the immediate weight-bearing forces. On AP pelvic radiographs identification of the iliopectineal line, the ilioischial line and the obturator fossa is essential. The iliopectineal line delineates the anterior column margin and the ilioischial line delineates the posterior column (Figure 5.14). The obturator fossa is involved in both columns. Traditionally, Judet views (45 degree oblique views) have been used to assess the anterior and posterior weight-bearing columns (Figure 5.15). The anterior wall of the acetabulum is smaller than the posterior wall and both are difficult to visualize on plain radiographs but are clearly demonstrated on CT.

There are a number of specific acetabular fracture patterns, which are frequently classified according to the Judet and Letournel system (Figure 5.16). This describes both simple and complex fracture patterns. The simple fractures are usually single injuries involving the anterior or posterior wall, anterior or posterior column or a simple transverse fracture. The more complex associated fracture types include combinations of injuries. Many of these occur in typical combination. For example posterior column and transverse fractures tend to fracture with the posterior wall. Delineation of fracture anatomy is essential for guiding surgeons as to the best stabilization technique. CT scanning is now routinely employed in acetabular fractures for further delineation of the fracture planes and associated pelvic injuries, to assess for the presence of a femoral head impaction fracture, the presence of loose bodies in the joint and for fractures of the anterior or posterior acetabular walls (Figure 5.17). Reformatted CT images are now being used to achieve similar display imaging to traditional oblique Judet views, thereby reducing patient disruption and reducing radiation exposure (Figure 5.18).

The evaluation of acetabular fractures can appear confusing and complex, but classification is possible with a few simple observations allowing quite accurate classification. If the obturator ring is disrupted there is a T-shaped or column fracture. The presence of

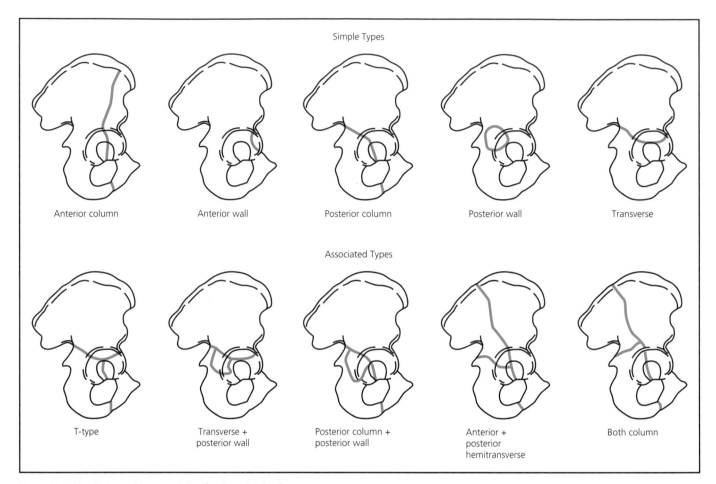

Figure 5.16 The Judet and Letournel classification of pelvic fractures.

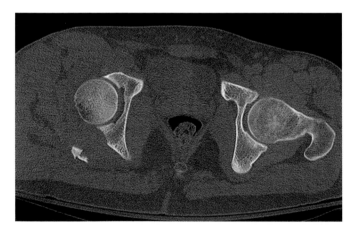

Figure 5.17 CT image demonstrating an isolated posterior wall fracture of the right acetabulum.

the spur sign, which is a strut of bone projected over the femoral head coming from the iliac blade, indicates a fracture of both columns and effective disconnection of this section of pelvis from the acetabulum (Figure 5.19). Disruption of the iliopectineal line on AP radiographs indicates anterior column injury, whereas dis-

ruption of the ilioischial line indicates posterior column injury. Disruption of both of these lines occurs in transverse and T-shaped fractures.

Acetabular fractures, while demanding expert assessment and treatment, are rarely early life-threatening complications of trauma.

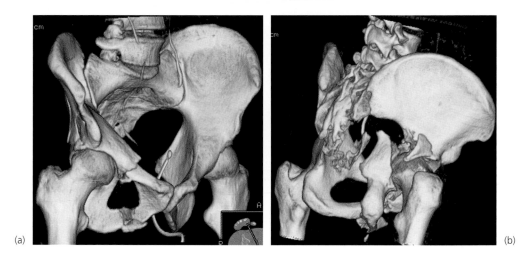

(a)

(b)

Figure 5.18 3D volume-rendered CT images of two patients with complex acetabular fractures involving both columns. (a) Right anterior oblique reformat simulating an obturator oblique Judet view, which demonstrates disruption of the anterior column; (b) posterior oblique reformat from a different patient demonstrates disruption of the posterior column.

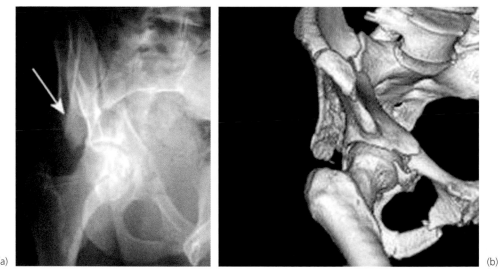

(a)

(b)

Figure 5.19 (a) Pelvic radiograph and (b) 3D CT scan demonstrating the spur sign (arrow) due to a strut of bone projecting from the sacroiliac joint to the lateral pelvic margin, which is caused by a fracture of both columns which effectively disconnects this section of pelvis from the acetabulum.

Complications tend to occur later with a major risk being post-traumatic osteoarthritis of the hip joint and sciatic nerve injury.

References

Brandser E and Marsh JL. Displaced acetabular fractures. *Clinical Orthopedics* 1988; **230:** 83–97.

Young JW, Burgess AR, Brumback RJ *et al.* Pelvic fractures: value of plain radiography in early assessment and management. *Radiology* 1986; **160:** 445–451.

Further reading

Dean Thornton D. Pelvic ring fractures. *eMedicine Radiology* 2007 (http://emedicine.medscape.com/article/394515-overview)

Mullins R. The influence of imaging on the trauma surgeon's evaluation of seriously injured patients. *Seminars in Roentgenology* 2006; **41:** 159–179.

Rogers LF. *Radiology of Skeletal Trauma.* Churchill Livingstone, Edinburgh, 2001.

Thacker MM, Tejwani N & Thakkar C. Acetabulum fractures. *eMedicine Orthopedics* 2008 (http://emedicine.com/orthoped/topic2.htm).

CHAPTER 6

Cervical Spine Trauma

Sivadas Ganeshalingam[1], Muaaze Ahmad[1], Evan Davies[2] and Leonard J. King[2]

[1]The Royal London Hospital, London, UK
[2]Southampton University Hospitals NHS Trust, Southampton, Hampshire, UK

OVERVIEW

- The cervical spine is frequently injured in major trauma
- Imaging is a useful adjunct to clinical evaluation in clearing the cervical spine
- Imaging of the cervical spine should not take priority over resuscitation procedures
- Multidetector computed tomography is an accurate means of demonstrating cervical spine fractures and is the imaging modality of choice in high-risk patients with major trauma
- Magnetic resonance imaging can be useful with neurological injury and to assess the intervertebral discs and ligaments
- Delays in clearing the cervical spine can result in increased morbidity due to aspiration, occipital pressure sores and raised intracranial pressure

Box 6.1 **Criteria for determining which patients do not require cervical spine imaging**

- Fully alert and orientated
- No head injury
- No drugs or alcohol
- No neck pain
- No abnormal neurology
- No significant distracting injury

(from the British Trauma Society guidelines)

Box 6.2 **High-risk parameters for cervical spine injury**

- High-velocity motor vehicle collision (>35mph)
- Death at scene of motor vehicle collision
- Fall >10 ft
- Closed head injury
- Fractures (pelvic, multiple limbs)
- Neurological symptoms or signs relating to the cervical spine

The majority of patients involved in major trauma require assessment of the cervical spine. Missed diagnosis of cervical spine injury can lead to severe neurological sequelae with 5–10% of neurological injuries resulting from delayed diagnosis and lack of appropriate cervical immobilization.

Who to image

According to British Trauma Society guidelines, clinical assessment can safely exclude spinal injury in patients who satisfy specific criteria (Box 6.1). If these criteria are fulfilled, there is no bruising, deformity or tenderness and a pain-free range of movement, then the cervical spine can be cleared clinically and radiological investigation is not indicated. Patients not fulfilling these criteria should be imaged.

How to image

The standard three-view plain film series (lateral, anteroposterior and open-mouth peg view) is an appropriate first-line investigation for blunt trauma in low-risk patients. Radiographs can be performed with the neck immobilized and the cervical collar in situ.

ABC of Imaging in Trauma. By Leonard J. King and David C. Wherry
Published 2010 by Blackwell Publishing

If the radiographs are normal, the patient is awake, alert with no neurology and has no persistent pain or tenderness they can be allowed to actively move the neck. It is unusual for clinically unsuspected fractures to be found on plain radiographs.

NICE guidelines advise that adult trauma patients who have any of the following criteria should undergo cervical spine computed tomography (CT):
- GCS below 13 on initial assessment
- intubation
- technically inadequate plain films
- suspicious or definitely abnormal radiographs
- patients being scanned for multitrauma.

High-risk patients (Box 6.2) should also undergo CT.

In the interpretation of multidetector computed tomography (MDCT) it is important to view thin-slice axial images plus coronal and sagittal reformats. The upper thoracic vertebral bodies are difficult to visualize on radiographs and cervical spine CT should be extended to the T4 vertebral body. The occipital condyles and the atlanto-occipital joints region should also be routinely viewed on

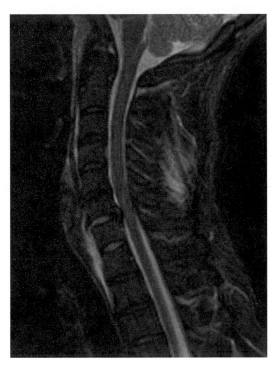

Figure 6.1 Sagittal short-tau inversion recovery (STIR) MR image demonstrating disruption of the anterior longitudinal ligament plus the C6/7 disc, posterior ligamentous oedema and cord contusion.

cervical CT and multiplaner reformats (MPRs) can be particularly useful for this.

The optimal method for clearing the cervical spine in obtunded trauma patients is controversial. An unequivocally normal, good-quality MDCT makes the presence of an unstable injury unlikely but may occasionally miss a purely soft tissue injury. Magnetic resonance imaging (MRI) can be used in this context to exclude a significant ligamentous injury but may be technically difficult to undertake in acute trauma patients who require close monitoring. MRI also demonstrates the presence of spinal cord compression, contusion, haemorrhage, acute disc prolapse or ligament damage following trauma (Figure 6.1) and is indicated in patients with neurological signs or suspicion of a disc or significant soft tissue injury.

The role of flexion/extension cervical radiographs

Lateral radiographs performed with the neck actively flexed and extended can be obtained to demonstrate ligament or disc injury in patients with normal radiographs or to demonstrate the stability of minor malalignments, which may be physiological or longstanding and due to pre-existing pathology. In the acute setting, however, the presence of instability may be underestimated due to muscle spasm, the cervicothoracic junction is often not visualized and there is a risk of acute neurological deterioration, thus these views are now less commonly employed.

Dynamic fluoroscopy of the cervical spine has been advocated by some centres but can be technically challenging, may miss unstable injuries, and carries a risk of neurological injury.

Anatomy of the cervical spine

The atlas – C1

The atlas is a ring structure consisting of two lateral articular masses plus an anterior and posterior arch (Figure 6.2a). The anterior tubercle arises from the anterior arch and articulates with the odontoid process of C2. A thin transverse process extends from each lateral articular mass and contains a notch or foramen through which the vertebral artery passes. The lateral articular masses have superior and inferior facets, which articulate with the occipital condyles above and the superior facets of the axis below.

The axis – C2

The axis (Figure 6.2b) has a vertebral body from which the odontoid process projects superiorly, sitting between the anterior arch of the atlas and the transverse ligament. The pedicles and laminae are relatively thick, and there is a wide central spinal canal. The transverse processes are small and perforated by the vertebral artery foramina. The large spinous process has a bifid tip.

C3–7 vertebrae

Each vertebra consists of an anterior body plus a posterior arch formed by two pedicles and laminae, which support seven processes; four articular facets, two transverse processes and a spinous process. Each vertebra articulates at the body and the superior plus inferior articular facets. The pedicles of these vertebral bodies are pierced at their base by the foramina transversaria, which transmit the vertebral arteries (except C7). The spinous processes are small and may have a bifid tip.

Upper cervical ligaments

Several ligaments provide support for the upper cervical spine, including the apical, alar and cruciate ligaments plus the tectorial membrane (Figure 6.3). The tectorial membrane is a broad continuation of the posterior longitudinal ligament extending between the posterior body of C2 and the basion, which limits extension at the atlanto-occipital joints. The alar ligaments are fan-shaped extending from the posterolateral odontoid to the inferomedial occipital condyles and the lateral masses of C1, which limit lateral tilt and rotation. The cruciate ligament consists of a superior crus, an inferior crus and the transverse ligament of the atlas, which attaches on the medial surface of the lateral masses of C1 and arches across the ring of the atlas posterior to the odontoid process.

Lower cervical ligaments

Several important ligaments help to support the mid and lower cervical spine, including the anterior longitudinal ligament, the posterior longitudinal ligament, capsular ligaments, interspinous ligaments, the suprasinous ligament and the ligamentum flavum. Stability of the cervical spine depends mainly on the anterior plus posterior longitudinal ligaments and the ligament flavum. These ligaments and the interspinous ligaments can be directly visualized on MRI.

The two-column concept of cervical spine stability

Cervical spine stability refers to the maintenance of satisfactory alignment under physiological loading without neurological compromise. Most imaging is performed without physiological

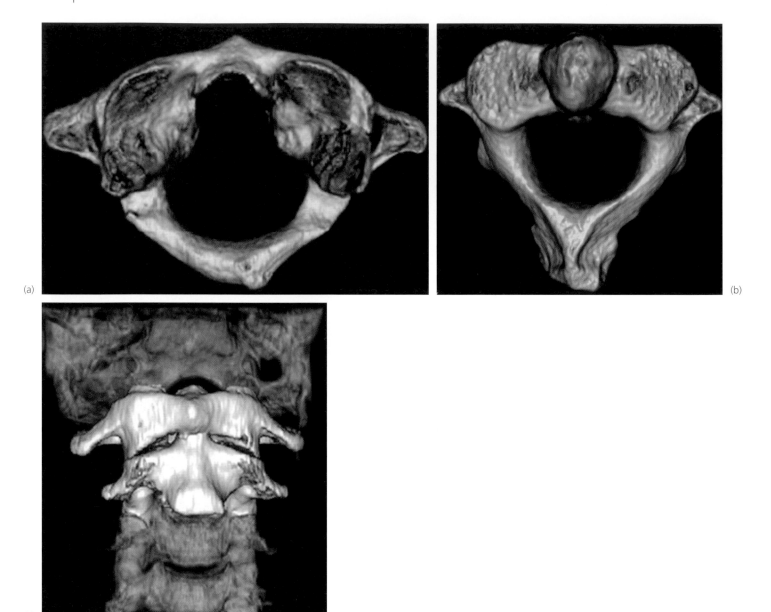

(a)

(b)

(c)

Figure 6.2 3D volume-rendered CT images of (a) C1 and (b) C2 viewed from above, and (c) C1 plus C2 viewed from the front demonstrating the normal anatomy and alignment.

loading, however, and there are no universally accepted criteria for assessing stability.

The subaxial spine can be evaluated using a two-column model (Figure 6.4). Cervical spines with an intact anterior column plus one intact posterior structure, or with an intact posterior column plus one intact anterior structure, remain biomechanically stable under physiological loads. Vertebral subluxations of greater than 2.7 mm (3.5 mm on radiographs) or acute kyphotic angulation of greater than 11 degrees are also associated with instability.

ABC interpretation of the lateral cervical spine radiograph

The lateral cervical spine radiograph is usually taken and examined before any other spinal films, although it has a false-negative rate of around 23%.

Adequacy: the lateral radiograph should demonstrate the occipito-cervical junction and all vertebrae down to the superior aspect of T1. The vertebrae should not be obscured by the shoulders or overlying objects such as jewellery.

Alignment: the anterior and posterior vertebral, spinolaminar and posterior spinous lines should be smooth, slightly lordotic and without any steps (Figure 6.5). Malalignment may be a sign of ligament injury or an occult fracture. The predental space between the posterior cortex of the C1 anterior arch and the anterior cortex of the dens should not measure more than 3 mm in adults and 5 mm in children.

A line drawn along the clivus should point to the dens and the basion-to-dens distance should be less than 12 mm. The posterior border of the foramen magnum should also line up with the spinolaminar line.

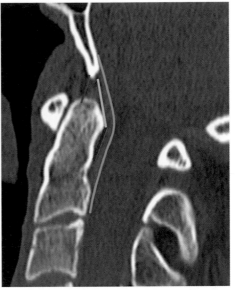

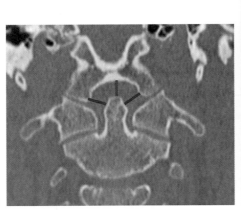

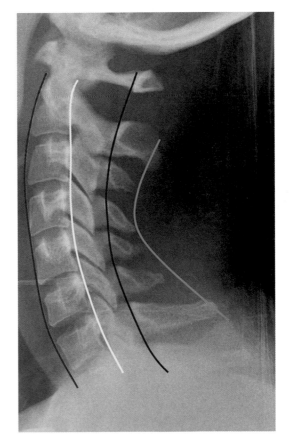

(a)   (b)

Figure 6.3 (a) Coronal and (b) sagittal CT reconstructions of the craniocervical junction with the upper cervical ligaments annotated (apical – blue, alar – red, superior crus of cruciate – orange, transverse – purple, tectorial membrane – green).

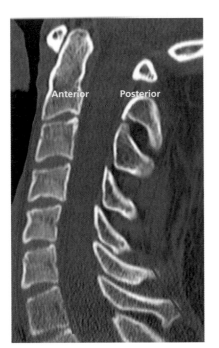

Anterior   Posterior

Figure 6.4 Sagittal CT reconstruction demonstrating the two column concept of cervical spine anatomy

- Anterior Column
  - ALL
  - Vertebral body
  - Intervertebral disc
  - PLL
  - Inter-transverse ligament
- Posterior Column
  - Laminae
  - Spinous process
  - Articular facets
  - Interspinous ligaments
  - Supraspinous ligament
  - Capsular ligaments
  - Ligamentum flavum

Figure 6.5 Lateral cervical spine radiograph demonstrating normal alignment of the anterior spinal line (red), posterior spinal line (yellow), spinolaminar line (blue) and the interspinous line (green).

Bone: the bony contour of each vertebral body should be traced. Posterior vertebral body height can be up to 3 mm more than the anterior vertebral body height. With dens fractures the C2 vertebra appears fatter than the C3 vertebra (fat C2 sign) and the normal C2 ring (Figure 6.6) is disrupted.

Cartilage: the disc spaces should be equal and symmetrical at all levels.

Soft tissue: the width and contour of the pre-vertebral soft tissues should be assessed. In the upper cervical spine from C2 to C4 the soft tissues should not exceed 7 mm or one-third of a vertebral body width, and below C4 should not exceed 21 mm or one vertebral body width. Widening of the soft tissues can be a useful indicator of injury, which may otherwise be radiographically occult. Absolute measurements are not an accurate indicator of injury,

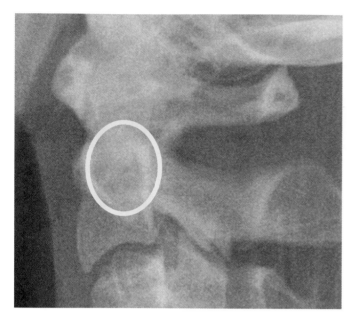

Figure 6.6 Lateral radiograph demonstrating a normal C2 ring.

however, and a normal pre-vertebral soft tissue pattern does not exclude injury. Loss of the normal soft tissue contour with localized bulging can also be a useful sign.

Interpretation of the anteroposterior radiograph

Adequacy: the spinous processes of all the cervical vertebrae from C2 to T1 should be visualized.

Alignment: the central spinous processes and the edges of the vertebral bodies and articular pillars should be aligned (Figure 6.7).

Bone: the cortical outline of each vertebral body should be smooth with no asymmetry in height or contour.

Cartilage: the cervical disc heights should be similar and symmetric but can be abnormal due to pre-existing degeneration.

Soft tissue: soft tissue swelling is usually less apparent on the anteroposterior (AP) view but surgical emphysema or foreign bodies may occasionally be demonstrated.

Interpretation of the open-mouth peg view

Adequacy: the entire odontoid peg and the lateral masses of C1 and C2 should be identified without rotation.

Alignment: the distance from the dens to the lateral masses should be equal on both sides and the lateral masses of C1 and C2 should be aligned (Figure 6.8).

Bone: the cortical margins should be smooth with no cortical breaks. Small notches are often present as a normal variant at the base of the odontoid peg.

Cartilage: the joint space between the inferior articular facets of C1 and the superior facets of C2 should be symmetrical.

Soft tissue: soft tissue swelling is not readily apparent on this projection.

Occipital condyle fractures

Occipital condyle fractures are markers of high-energy trauma that are associated with traumatic brain and cervical spine injuries.

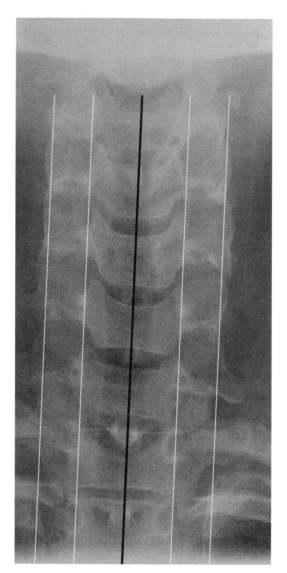

Figure 6.7 Anteroposterior radiograph of the cervical spine demonstrating normal spinous process and articular pillar alignment.

They are poorly demonstrated by conventional radiographs and are now increasingly diagnosed in survivors of high-energy blunt trauma due to widespread use of CT (Figure 6.9). They are important to recognize as there may be associated instability of the occipito-atlanto-axial joint complex. The integrity of this complex articulation is dependent on several supporting ligaments, of which the tectorial membrane and alar ligaments are the most important. Fractures at the insertions of these ligaments are equivalent to intrinsic disruptions and occipital condyle fractures may therefore lead to craniocervical junction instability.

The most widely used radiologic classification was described by Anderson and Montesano (Table 6.1). Type III injuries are the most common and may be associated with disruption of the alar ligaments and tectorial membrane resulting in craniocervical dissociation. A more recent classification by Tuli *et al.* (Table 6.2) may help to guide neurosurgical management with Type 1 injuries requiring no specific treatment, Type 2A injuries requiring treatment with a rigid collar and Type 2B fractures requiring surgical

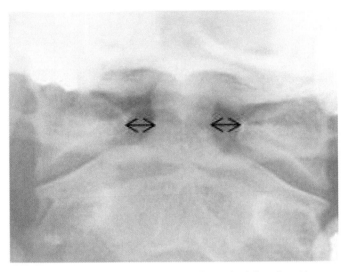

Figure 6.8 Open-mouth anteroposterior radiograph of the odontoid process demonstrating normal alignment. The distance from the dens to the C1 lateral masses should be symmetrical (arrows) and the tips of the lateral masses of C1 should line up with the lateral margins of the superior articular facets.

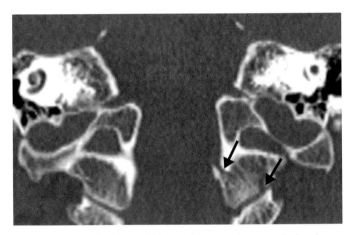

Figure 6.9 Coronal reformat CT image demonstrating an undisplaced impaction fracture of the left occipital condyle (arrows).

Table 6.1 Anderson and Montesano classification of occipital condyle fractures

Type	Description	Biomechanics
I	Impaction	Axial loading Ipsilateral alar ligament may be compromised Stability maintained by contralateral alar ligament and tectorial membrane
II	Skull base extension	Extends from occipital bone via condyle to foramen magnum Stability maintained by intact alar ligaments and tectorial membrane
III	Avulsion	Alar ligament avulsion Associated disruption of tectorial membrane and contralateral alar ligament may cause instability

Table 6.2 Classification of occipital condyle fractures (Tuli *et al.*)

Type	Description	Biomechanics
1	Non-displaced	Stable
2A	Displaced[a]	Stable; no radiographic, CT or MR imaging evidence of occipito-atlanto-axial instability or ligamentous disruption
2B	Displaced[a]	Unstable; positive radiographic, CT or MR imaging evidence of occipito-atlanto-axial instability or ligamentous disruption

[a]Defined as presence of at least 2 mm osseous separation.

instrumentation or halo traction. CT cannot reliably show disruption of the tectorial membrane and alar ligaments, which requires MRI assessment.

Injuries to the C1/C2 complex

Around 19–25% of cervical spine fractures involve the C1/2 complex. The unique anatomical relationship between the atlas and axis produces a variety of injury patterns not seen elsewhere in the spine. Numerous developmental anomalies that can mimic injury also occur, including:

- failure of fusion or absence of the anterior arch of C1 and the posterior arches of C1 or C2
- hypoplasia of the dens
- accessory ossicles including os terminale at the tip of the dens
- an ossicle adjacent to the anterior arch of C1
- primary spondylolisthesis of C2
- assimilation of C1 into the occiput.

Os odontoideum is due to a previous fracture of the odontoid process synchondrosis and causes instability, whereas ossiculum terminale is due to failure of fusion of the secondary ossification centre.

CT is particularly useful for accurately assessing C1/C2 injuries, occasionally supplemented by dynamic CT in cases of rotatory fixation.

Atlas fractures (Table 6.3)
Fracture of posterior elements of C1
The commonest type of atlas fracture is disruption of the posterior arch due to compression between the occiput and the posterior arch of the axis on hyperextension.

Jefferson fracture
First reported by Sir Geoffrey Jefferson in 1920, this fracture is due to axial loading with compression of the lateral masses between the occipital condyles and articular facets of C2. Fractures involve the anterior plus posterior arches of C1 and may be unilateral or bilateral, resulting in two, three or four fracture fragments. The classic four-part Jefferson fracture consists of bilateral disruption of the anterior and posterior arches with lateral displacement of both lateral masses (Figure 6.10). The transverse ligament is intact and the injury is stable.

Table 6.3 Gehweiler classification of atlas fractures

Classification	Mechanism of injury	Stability
I – Isolated bony apophysis fracture (extra-articular fracture of transverse process)		Stable. May involve vertebral foramen/artery
II – Isolated posterior arch fracture	Hyperextension	Stable
III – Isolated anterior arch fracture	Hyperextension Dens forced anteriorly through the C1 anterior arch	Unstable if displaced
IV – Comminuted lateral mass fracture	Lateral axial compression	Unstable
V – Burst fracture, three or more fragments	Axial compression	Depends on displacement/integrity of transverse ligament

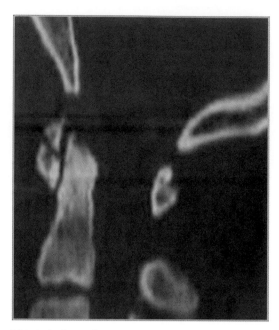

Figure 6.11 Sagittal CT reformat image demonstrating a horizontal fracture through the anterior arch of C1.

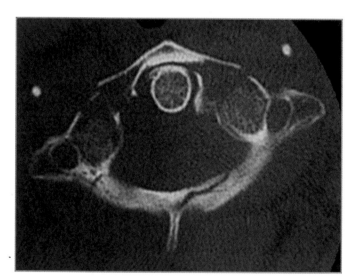

Figure 6.10 Axial CT image of C1 demonstrating a four-part Jefferson fracture.

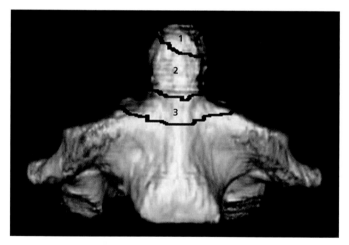

Figure 6.12 3D volume-rendered CT image demonstrating the Anderson and D'Alonzo classification of odontoid process fractures.

Type 1	Oblique fracture through upper part of the odontoid due to avulsion of alar ligament. Stable, high rate of fusion
Type 2	Fracture at junction of odontoid process and body of C2. Unstable, high rate of malunion
Type 3	Fracture extending down into body of C2. Stable, with high rate of fusion

Plough fracture

This is a rare fracture due to hyperextension at the craniocervical junction. There are usually bilateral vertical fractures of the anterior arch of C1 with anterior displacement of the comminuted fragment, which remains in articulation with the odontoid process.

Horizontal fractures of the anterior arch of C1

This is a rare fracture due to hyperextension. The pull of the anterior longitudinal ligament results in an avulsion fracture of the mid-portion of the anterior arch of the atlas (Figure 6.11).

Axis fractures
Fracture of the odontoid process

These fractures account for >50% of C2 fractures and are due to combination of extreme flexion, extension or rotation, along with

a shearing force. The Anderson and D'Alonzo classification (Figure 6.12) has therapeutic and prognostic implications. Between 31 and 65% of dens fractures are Type 2 (Figure 6.13) and are complicated by non-union in 26–36% of cases.

Hangman's fracture

This is a traumatic spondylolisthesis due to bilateral pars interarticularis fractures, which accounts for 4–23% of cervical spine frac-

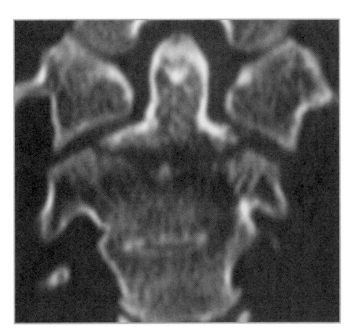

Figure 6.13 Coronal CT reformat demonstrating a Type 3 fracture of the odontoid process

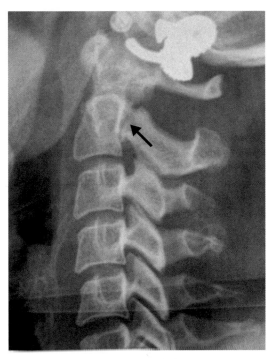

Figure 6.14 Lateral cervical spine radiograph demonstrating a type 1 hangman's fracture of C2 (arrow).

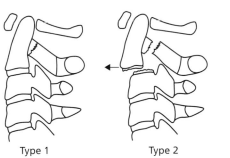
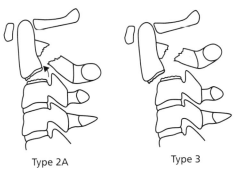

| Type 1 | Type 2 | Type 2A | Type 3 |

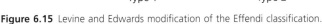

Figure 6.15 Levine and Edwards modification of the Effendi classification.

Type 1   Non-angulated, undisplaced or minimally displaced (<2–3 mm) with a normal disc at C2/C3
Type 2   Anteriorly displaced fracture of C2
Type 2A   Significant angulation without marked translation (PLL disrupted)
Type 3   Anterior displacement and hyperflexion of the axis in association with unilateral or bilateral C2/C3 facet dislocation

tures (Figure 6.14). The neural arch of C2 is avulsed from the C2 vertebral body due to vertical compression and hyperextension similar to the osseous injury produced by judicial hanging. The odontoid process remains intact. It is critical to differentiate between Type 2 and Type 2A fractures as traction is an appropriate treatment for Type 2 but not Type 2A fractures (Figure 6.15).

Extension teardrop fracture

This injury most commonly occurs at C2 and is due to hyperextension with avulsion of the anteroinferior corner of the vertebral body by the attached anterior longitudinal ligament (Figure 6.16). The vertical height of the fracture fragment is usually greater than its horizontal width.

Other axis fractures

Additional fractures of C2 include oblique vertebral body fractures and isolated fractures of the pedicle, lateral mass, lamina or spinous process.

Atlanto-axial subluxation

Post-traumatic atlanto-axial subluxation is rare. Subluxation results after tearing of the transverse ligament or avulsion fractures at the insertions of the transverse ligament.

Atlanto-axial rotatory fixation

This entity is a persistant pathological fixation of the atlanto-axial joint in a rotated position such that the atlas and the axis move as

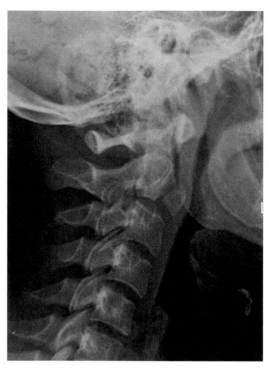

Figure 6.16 Lateral cervical spine radiograph demonstrating an extension teardrop fracture of C2.

> Box 6.3 **Fielding and Hawkins' classification of atlanto-axial rotatory fixation**
>
> I <3 mm anterior displacement of atlas on axis with intact transverse ligament
> II 3–5 mm anterior displacement with deficient transverse ligament
> III >5 mm anterior displacement of atlas on axis with deficient transverse and secondary ligaments
> IV posterior displacement of atlas on axis

a single unit rather than independently. The Fielding and Hawkins classification system is based on the direction and degree of displacement, Type 1 being the most common injury and Type 4 the least common (Box 6.3).

Complex atlanto-axial fractures

Fractures involving both C1 and C2 are relatively common but less frequent than isolated C1 and C2 fractures. The commonest pattern of injury is an odontoid process fracture with interruption of the anterior and/or posterior arch of C1.

Fractures of the 3rd to 7th cervical vertebrae

There are numerous fracture patterns in the mid/lower cervical spine resulting from a combination of flexion, hyperextension and rotational forces.

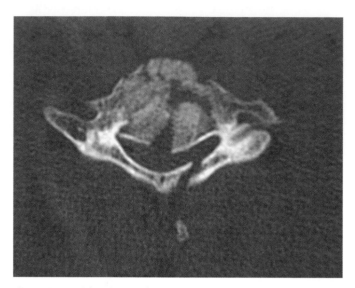

Figure 6.17 Axial CT image of a C7 burst fracture with retropulsed fragments narrowing the spinal canal.

Compression fractures

These fractures result from vertical loading with loss of vertebral body height, disruption of the anterior cortex and depression of the superior end plate. They are usually stable injuries and typically do not cause neural compromise. CT is useful to evaluate the posterior elements and ensure that there is no posterior wall retropulsion.

Burst fractures

Burst fractures are due to axial compression and in contrast to compression fractures there is loss of height of the anterior and posterior vertebral body. They usually occur in the lower cervical spine. There is retropulsion of posterior wall fragments into the spinal canal, which can result in cord damage. CT is useful to assess the degree of retropulsion and spinal canal narrowing (Figure 6.17). MRI is also useful to demonstrate associated epidural haematoma and cord injury. These fractures are unstable as there is damage to both the anterior and posterior columns.

Flexion teardrop fracture

This is a major injury resulting from hyperflexion and compression with distraction of the posterior elements. There is a teardrop-shaped fracture fragment arising from the antero-inferior aspect of the vertebral body, most commonly at C5 (Figure 6.18). The vertebral body may be subluxed, which can compromise the spinal canal, and CT is indicated to assess for the degree of retropulsion. The spinous processes may also be fractured and there is associated ligament and disc injury. These injuries should be considered unstable.

Unilateral facet subluxation/dislocation

This injury is due to rotation and flexion with rupture of the apophyseal ligaments and is often stable. On lateral cervical radiographs the facet joints do not align correctly. There is a gradation of injury from minor subluxation to perched facets and severe-locked facets (Figure 6.19). With locked facets there is a bat wings appearance on CT due to the facets only partially overlapping. There is usually also anterior subluxation of the involved vertebral body by less than 50% of the vertebral body width. On AP radio-graphs there is a sudden change in the spinous process alignment with the spinous process above the injury rotated towards the involved side. There may be associated fractures of the articular facets. Isolated facet fractures can also occur without associated subluxation.

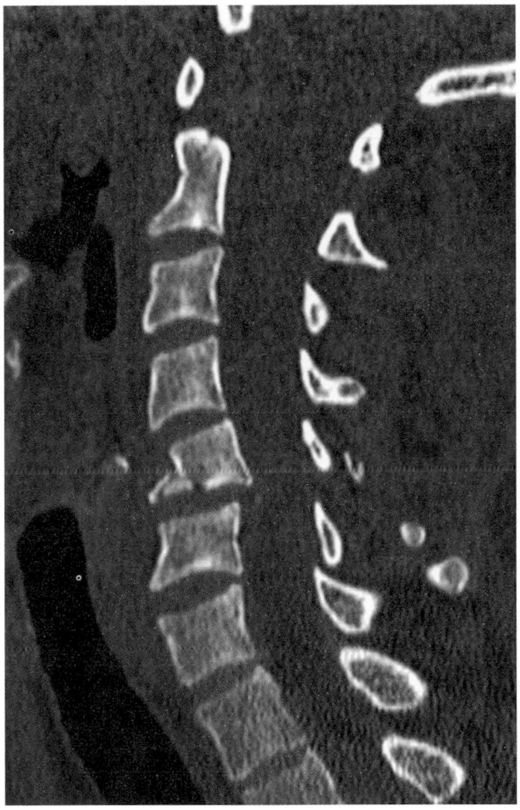

Bilateral facet subluxation/dislocation

This is due to hyperflexion injury and usually causes anterior vertebral subluxation greater than 50% of the vertebral body width, in addition to the variable degree of facet joint displacement (Figure 6.20). These are unstable injuries, which have a high risk of associated spinal cord damage, although typically there are no fractures of the facets. On AP radiographs the vertical alignment of the spinous processes remains normal but there is abnormal widening of the inter-spinous distance. CT and MRI can be useful to assess the full extent of this injury.

Transverse process fractures

These fractures are common and may involve the foramen transversarium (Figure 6.21). The vertebral artery is therefore at risk and contrast-enhanced CT is useful to exclude vascular injury.

Lamina fractures

Fractures of the laminae may occur in isolation, as part of a lateral mass fracture or a more complex injury such as a flexion teardrop injury. Isolated fractures are regarded as stable.

Spinous process fractures

Fractures of the lower cervical spinous processes are known as a "clay shoveler's" fracture (Figure 6.22). These characteristically occur at C6–T1 and are due to a hyperflexion injury. These are stable injuries, which are usually evident on lateral radiographs. An associated laminar or facet fracture should be excluded with CT.

Figure 6.18 Sagittal CT reformat of a C5 flexion teardrop injury.

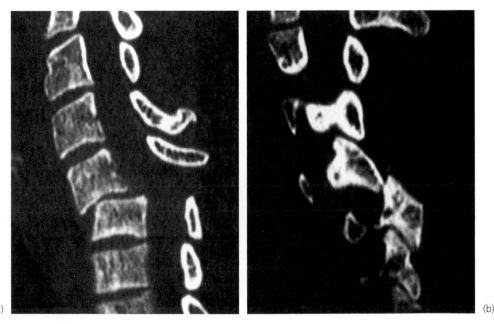

(a) (b)

Figure 6.19 (a) Midline sagittal and (b) parasagittal CT reformats demonstrating a unifacet dislocation at C5/6.

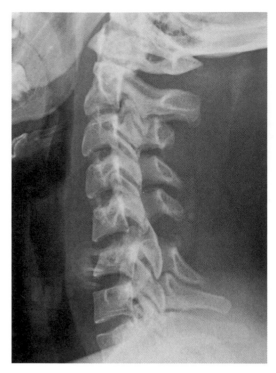

Figure 6.20 Lateral radiograph of a bilateral facet subluxation. The vertebral subluxation is less than 50% in this case.

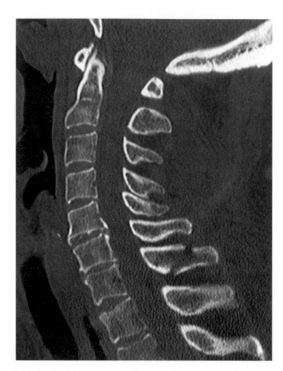

Figure 6.22 Sagittal CT reformat of a C7 spinous process fracture.

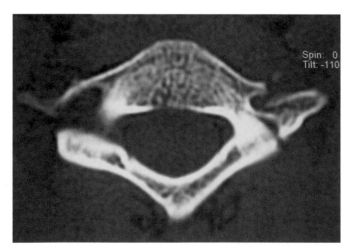

Figure 6.21 Axial CT image of a left transverse process fracture.

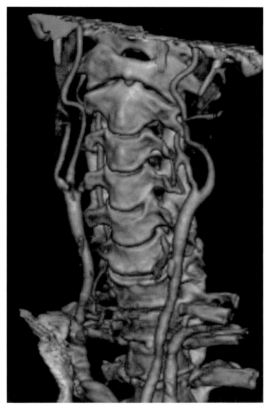

Figure 6.23 Volume rendered reformats of the cervical spine demonstrating occlusion of the left vertebral artery.

Vascular injury

Vascular injury is typically under-diagnosed in the setting of acute cervical trauma. The vertebral arteries are closely related to the cervical spine; they are at particular risk in trauma and are frequently injured. The vertebral artery enters at the C6 transverse foramen and extends vertically from C6 to C1. This segment of the vertebral artery is most at risk from trauma, particularly from transverse foramen fractures. In patients with unexplained neurological clinical features such as hemiparesis, dysphagia, Horner's syndrome or transient ischaemic attack, a vascular injury should be excluded. The diagnosis of vascular injury can be made by contrast enhanced CT, MRI or catheter angiography (Figure 6.23).

Brachial plexus

The brachial plexus can be injured by stretching or tearing of the nerve roots due to blunt trauma or by direct injury from penetrating trauma. Injuries vary in severity from a first-degree neuropraxia to complete nerve transaction. Lesions are classified as post- or pre-ganglionic. Pre-ganglionic injuries are either central avulsions from the spinal cord or intradural rootlet ruptures proximal to the dorsal root ganglion. MRI can be useful to assess these lesions particularly to demonstrate pre-ganglionic injury, which is not amenable to surgical repair.

Further reading

CG56 Head Injury, NICE guideline September 2007.

Cassar-Pullicino VN & Imhof H. Spinal trauma – an imaging approach.

Hanson JA, Blackmore CC, Mann FA & Wilson AJ. Cervical spine injury: a clinical decision rule to identify high-risk patients for helical CT screening. *American Journal of Roentgenology* 2000; **174**: 713–717.

Harris TJ, Blackmore CC, Mirza SK & Jurkovich GJ. Clearing the cervical spine in obtunded patients. *Spine* 2008; **33**:1547–1553.

Hogan GJ, Mirvis SE, Shanmuganathan K & Scalea TM. Exclusion of cervical spine injury in obtunded patients with blunt trauma: is MR imaging needed when multidetector row CT findings are normal? *Radiology* 2005; **237**:106–113.

Oakley P, Brohi K, Wilson A *et al*. Guidelines for initial management and assessment of spinal injury. British Trauma Society, 2002. *Injury* 2003; **34**: 405–425.

Tins BJ & Cassar-Pullicino VN. Imaging of acute cervical spine injuries: review and outlook. *Clinical Radiology* 2004; **59**: 865–880.

Van Goethem J, Maes M, Ozsarlak O *et al*. Imaging in spinal trauma. *European Radiology* 2005; **15**: 582–590.

CHAPTER 7

Thoracic and Lumbar Spine Trauma

Sivadas Ganeshalingam[1], Muaaze Ahmad[1], Evan Davies[2] and Leonard J. King[2]

[1]The Royal London Hospital, London, UK
[2]Southampton University Hospitals NHS Trust, Southampton, Hampshire, UK

OVERVIEW

- Spinal immobilization is a priority in multiple trauma patients but clearance is not
- Imaging of the spine does not take precedence over life-saving procedures
- Fractures of the thoracolumbar spine can be stable or unstable
- Whole-body multidetector computed tomography gives high-quality images of the thoracic and lumbar spine
- Magnetic resonance imaging can be useful in selected cases following trauma particularly when there are abnormal neurological signs

Significant trauma is usually required to injure the thoracolumbar spine, which is less mobile and better supported by surrounding anatomical structures than the cervical spine. Injuries can occur in isolation but are frequently encountered in polytrauma victims and typically arise from motor vehicle collisions, sports activities or falls, with the thoracolumbar junction at particular risk. Penetrating injuries to the spine are also occasionally encountered (Figure 7.1).

Who to image

The current standard for radiological evaluation of the thoracolumbar spine is not clearly defined and the decision to image will depend on the individual clinical scenario. British Trauma Society guidelines advise that imaging is clearly indicated if there is pain, bruising, swelling, deformity or abnormal neurology which can be determined on clinical evaluation in alert, conscious patients, with no major distracting injuries. Clinical assessment is often incomplete or misleading, however, due to altered consciousness or distracting injury. Unconscious patients with a significant mechanism of injury should undergo imaging of the whole spine.

There should be a high index of suspicion in patients who:
- have fallen from a height
- are unconscious with multiple injuries
- have neurological symptoms or signs, or radiological evidence of fractures to the posterior ribs, scapula, sternum or calcaneum.

Patients with underlying conditions such as known spinal malignancy, osteoporosis, degenerative disease, ankylosing spondylitis, previous fusion or congenital anomalies have an increased risk of injury and a higher index of suspicion is necessary.

Patients with one fracture of the thoracolumbar spine have a 5–15% overall risk of a second fracture, which may be discontinuous. This risk rises to around 40% in patients with burst fractures, and thus detection of one fracture should lead to evaluation of the entire spine for concomitant injuries.

How to image

Anteroposterior (AP) and lateral radiographs are an appropriate first line investigation for patients with isolated spine injury, proceeding to computed tomography (CT) for further evaluation of potentially unstable injuries, poorly demonstrated areas or equivocal lesions.

Polytrauma patients undergoing multidetector computed tomography (MDCT) of the torso do not routinely require radiographs of the spine as the CT data can be reformatted with a bony algorithm and small field of view to give detailed images with a high sensitivity for injuries. Additional erect radiographs are sometimes required by spinal surgeons to help assess the stability of injuries that may be suitable for non-operative management.

Magnetic resonance imaging (MRI) is indicated in the presence of neurological symptoms or signs which may localize to the spinal cord or cauda equina in order to assess the extent of injury and ongoing neural compression (Figure 7.2). MRI is also particularly useful for demonstrating ligament injury, acute traumatic disc herniation, epidural haematoma, cord transaction, radiographically occult vertebral body fractures (Figure 7.3) and spinal cord injury without radiographic abnormality (SCIWORA). Cord oedema has a relatively favourable outcome compared with cord haemorrhage, and these may be distinguished on MR imaging thus providing useful prognostic information.

Anatomy of vertebral bodies

There are twelve thoracic and five lumbar vertebrae, often with normal variation at the lumbar sacral junction, including a transitional vertebral body or incomplete fusion of the posterior elements. Each vertebrae comprises of a body and spinous process

ABC of Imaging in Trauma. By Leonard J. King and David C. Wherry
Published 2010 by Blackwell Publishing

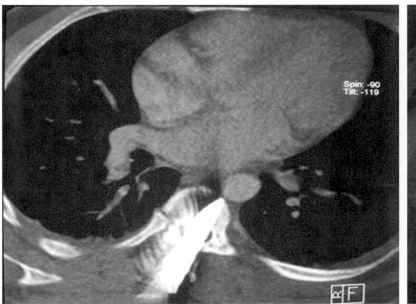

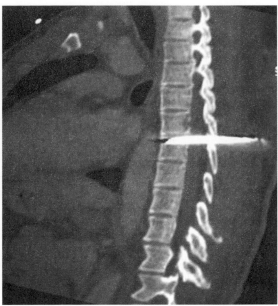

(a)　　　　　　　　　　　　　　　　　　　　　　　　　　　　　　　　(b)

Figure 7.1 (a) Axial and (b) sagittal CT reconstruction of the thoracic spine demonstrating a knife injury.

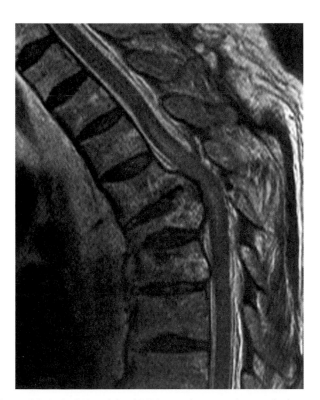

Figure 7.2 Sagittal T2 weighted MR image demonstrating vertebral fractures at three contiguous levels and oedema in the mid-thoracic cord.

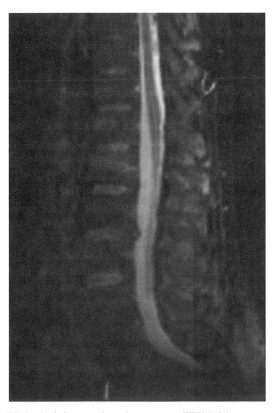

Figure 7.3 Sagittal short-tau inversion recovery (STIR) MR image demonstrating radiographically occult compression fractures at T12 and L1 in a pilot following ejection from a jet fighter.

plus two paired pedicles, transverse processes, superior and inferior articular facets, pars interarticularis and laminae. In the thoracic spine there are articular facets on the lateral aspect of the vertebral bodies for articulation with the ribs. The lumbar vertebral bodies are larger and have a horizontal spinous process. There are numerous ligaments that support the spine, including the anterior and posterior longitudinal ligaments, the ligamentum flavum the inter-

spinous ligaments and the supraspinous ligament. The paraspinal muscles also provide support.

The thoracic spinal canal is narrow in relation to the spinal cord, which is therefore at risk of injury. The spinal cord ends at around

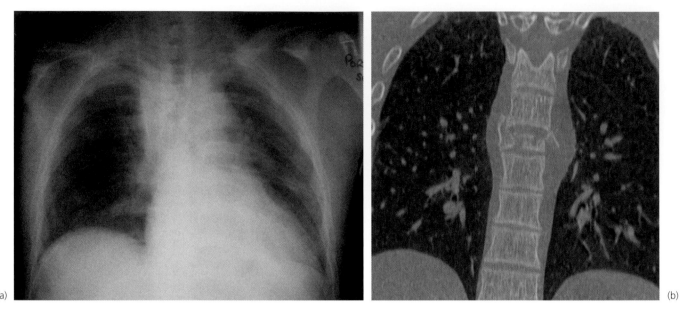

(a)   (b)

Figure 7.4 Widening of the paraspinal soft tissues on (a) a chest radiograph and (b) coronal CT reformat image in two patients with thoracic spine fractures.

the L1 level and fractures below this level tend to be less significant neurologically with relatively greater space for the lower motor neurone roots of the cauda equina.

ABC Assessment of the thoracic and lumbar radiograph

Adequacy/alignment: the thoracic and lumbar vertebrae should all be visualized on both the lateral and AP radiographs with sufficient penetration to visualize the pedicles. There should be a gentle mid-thoracic kyphosis and lumbar lordosis. The anterior and posterior longitudinal lines should be smooth. The distance between the pedicles on the frontal radiograph should not vary by more than 2 mm from one level to another.

Bones: the vertebral bodies should show a slight sequential increase in height extending caudally and be of similar height anteriorly and posteriorly with no more than a 2 mm discrepancy, except at T11–L1 where slight anterior wedging can be a normal finding. The outline of each vertebral body, pedicle, transverse and spinous process should be traced.

Cartilage: the inter-vertebral disc spaces should be similar throughout the thoracic spine and increase in size caudally in the lumbar region, with L4/5 disc being the widest. The presence of degenerative disc disease causes reduction of the inter-vertebral distance.

Soft tissues: in the thorax a displaced para-spinal line indicates pathology and in the traumatic setting a vertebral body fracture (Figure 7.4) is likely. In the abdomen loss of the psoas shadow may indicate a retroperitoneal haematoma.

Injury patterns

Most adult injuries occur at the thoracolumbar junction (T11–L2) due to relative mobility and loss of the protective effects of the ribs at this point. The main mechanisms of thoracolumbar spine

Box 7.1 **Mechanisms of thoracolumbar spine injury**

- Flexion
- Flexion distraction
- Flexion rotation
- Axial load
- Fracture dislocation
- Shearing (Translation)
- Hyperextension

trauma are flexion, compression, distraction and rotational injury (Box 7.1). Multiple force vectors often occur in combination, however, such as flexion and axial loading, thus limiting accurate classification based on mechanism of injury.

Injuries to the thoracolumbar spine can be minor or major. Minor injuries include transverse process (Figure 7.5), spinous process, pars interarticularis and isolated articular process fractures, which can be considered stable. Major injuries range from relatively simple anterior compression injuries to complex fracture dislocations with gross instability. Classification of these injuries is difficult and controversial. Denis developed a three-column model of spinal stability based on imaging findings, dividing the spine into anterior, middle and posterior columns (Figure 7.6). Disruption of either two or three columns, or the middle column indicates that an injury is unstable. The Denis system may oversimplify complex fractures however, and may not accurately assess the need for operative intervention.

The AO classification of thoracolumbar fractures is now being commonly used by spinal surgeons. It divides fractures into a total of 53 potential patterns based on three injury types – A, B and C (Box 7.2) – each of which contains three subgroups with specifications. The classification reflects a progressive scale of

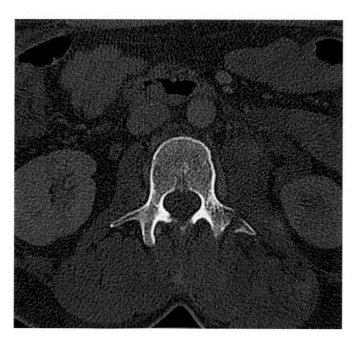

Figure 7.5 Axial CT image demonstrating a minor fracture of a left-sided lumbar transverse process.

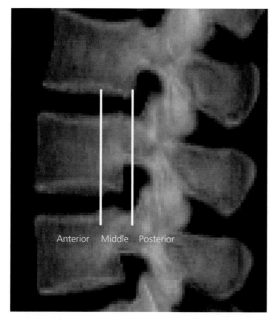

Figure 7.6 The three-column anatomy of the thoracic and lumbar spine. Anterior column – anterior vertebral body, anterior annulus fibrosus, anterior longitudinal ligament. Middle column – posterior vertebral body, posterior longitudinal ligament, posterior annulus fibrosus. Posterior column – posterior bony elements, ligament flavum, posterior ligaments.

morphological damage by which the degree of instability is determined. Categories are established according to the main mechanism of injury, pathomorphological uniformity and in consideration of prognostic aspects regarding healing potential. The types have a fundamental injury pattern, which is determined by the three most

> **Box 7.2 Thoracolumbar fracture types according to the AO classification of injuries**
>
> - Type A – Vertebral body compression
> - Type B – Anterior and posterior element injury with distraction
> - Type C – Anterior and posterior element injury with rotation

important mechanisms acting on the spine: compression, distraction and axial torque. Morphological criteria are predominantly used for further subdivision of the injuries. Severity progresses from Type A to Type C, as well as within the types, groups and further subdivisions. The use of all 53 different fracture patterns is rather unwieldy, however, and system has poor inter- and intra-observer agreement other than for the main types.

Compression fractures

These are flexion compression injuries often involving only the anterior column. They can involve the superior end plate, the inferior end plate, both end plates or the anterior cortex with intact end plates. They are generally considered to be stable and typically have no associated neurological deficit (Figure 7.7). These fractures may extend to the posterior wall, however, and with increasing loss of anterior vertebral body height there is an increased likelihood of posterior ligamentous injury, thus these injuries can be unstable (Figure 7.8).

Compression fractures can be clearly demonstrated on good-quality lateral radiographs with reduced anterior vertebral body height and preservation of the posterior vertebral body height. The alignment is often relatively well maintained, although there may be a degree of acute kyphotic deformity. MDCT can be useful to exclude any concomitant spinal injury and to assess the posterior wall and spinal canal.

Burst fractures

Burst fractures are often due to falling from a height, producing vertical compression force. Injuries usually occur from T4 to L5, most commonly at L1, often in association with calcaneal or pelvic fractures. The intervertebral disc is driven down into the vertebral body causing a comminuted fracture, which disrupts the anterior and middle columns. The posterior elements may also be involved. Fragments from the posterior wall are retropulsed into the spinal canal and may compress the cord or cauda equina (Figure 7.9).

Burst fractures can be both stable and unstable injuries depending on the severity of the injury pattern. If the posterior column is involved it is an unstable injury. If there is fracture dislocation, loss of more than 50% of vertebral body height or more than 20% angulation at the thoracolumbar junction an unstable injury is present. A significant fracture is typically associated with posterior ligament complex injury and/ or facet joint injury.

On spine radiographs there is usually a vertical fracture of the vertebral body with loss of anterior and posterior body height and widening of the interpedicular distance (Figure 7.10). The posterior wall may also be indistinct or obviously retropulsed. CT should

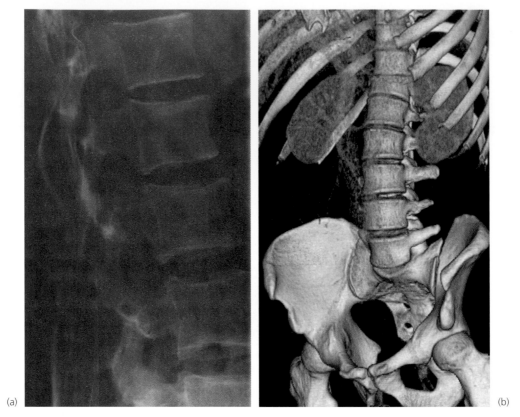

(a)   (b)

Figure 7.7 (a) Lateral radiograph of the lumbar spine demonstrating minor anterior wedge compression fractures at T12 and L1; (b) 3D volume-rendered reconstruction from a different patient demonstrating a kyphotic deformity at T12 due to a compression fracture.

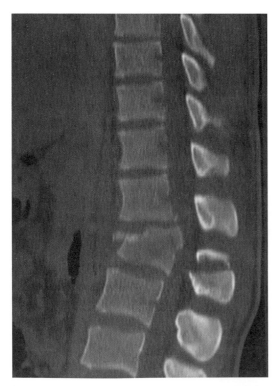

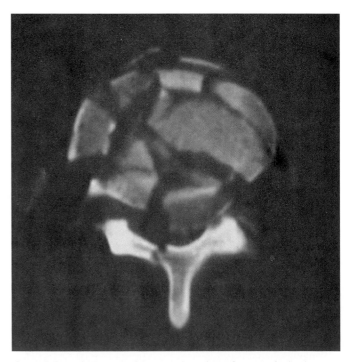

Figure 7.9 Axial CT image demonstrating a burst fracture of a lumbar vertebral body with retropulsed fragments in the spinal canal.

Figure 7.8 Sagittal CT reconstruction demonstrating an unstable thoracic spine hyperflexion injury with disruption of the anterior, middle and posterior columns.

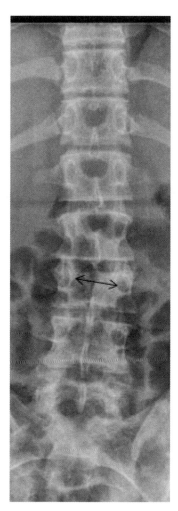

Figure 7.10 Anteroposterior radiograph of the lumbar spine demonstrating widening of the interpedicular distance due to a compression fracture.

Box 7.3 **Characteristic features of Chance type flexion-distraction injuries**

- Disruption of posterior elements (osseous/ligamentous)
- Widening of posterior elements
- Minimal or no loss of anterior vertebral body height
- Minimal or no anterior displacment of the vertebral body or the superior vertebral body fragment
- Minimal or no lateral displacement of the vertebral body or the superior vertebral body fragment
- Posterior vertebral body height equal or greater than the vertebral body below

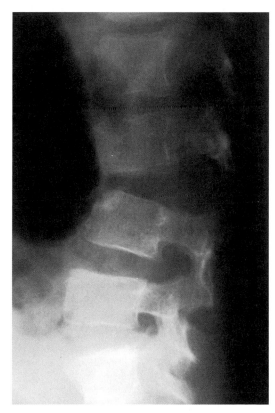

Figure 7.11 Lateral radiograph of a child with a flexion distraction injury disrupting the posterior ligaments and the intervertebral disc.

be performed to assess the spinal canal for retropulsed fragments and associated posterior element injury.

Flexion distraction injuries

There are several variations on this injury pattern, which usually occurs at a single level from L1 to L3 due to horizontal cleavage forces, often resulting from motor vehicle collisions with a lap belt restraint. These injuries are all unstable.

The chance fracture is the commonest type of flexion distraction injury typically occurring at the L1–3 levels (Box 7.3). A horizontal plane fracture extends from the involved posterior elements (laminae, pedicles and spinous process) into the posterosuperior portion of the vertebral body. There is typically no significant anterior compression and the interspinous ligament is spared. The Smith fracture is a similar horizontal plane fracture, which spares the spinous process and instead involves the interspinous ligament, which is disrupted with widening of the interspinous distance. A unilateral variant of the flexion distraction injury pattern is also described secondary to a rotational force. The anterior longitudinal ligament is not usually involved. Flexion distraction injury can also disrupt the intervertebral disc rather than the vertebral body, giving rise to subluxation and a higher incidence of neurological injury (Figure 7.11).

Lateral radiographs can demonstrate the horizontal fractures and AP films the transverse clefts in the pedicles and spinous processes. The "empty vertebral body" sign with lack of overlap between the vertebral body and posterior elements may also be demonstrated due to elevation of the posterior elements. The extent of the bony injury is best appreciated on sagittal CT reconstructions; however, MRI allows accurate assessment of ligamentous structures such as the anterior and posterior longitudinal ligaments, the

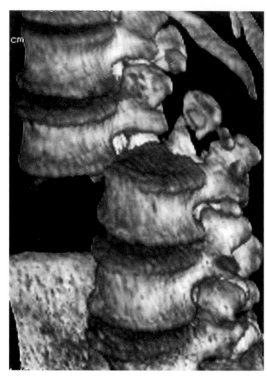

Figure 7.12 Surface shaded 3D CT reformat image demonstrating a severe fracture dislocation at L2/3.

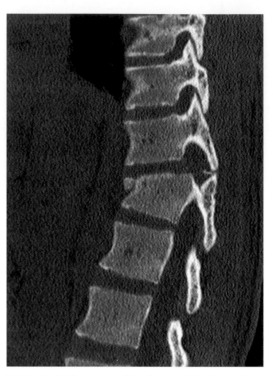

Figure 7.13 Sagittal CT reconstruction of an unstable three-column hyperflexion injury with subluxation and perching of the facet joints.

interspinous ligament, the supraspinous ligament and the ligamentum flavum, as well any associated spinal cord injury.

Fracture-dislocation

Fracture dislocation injuries are usually due to a combination of force vectors. There is displacement of one vertebra with respect to another, usually with an associated fracture producing disruption of all three columns, and they are thus highly unstable, often with associated neurological injury. There are numerous different injury patterns that can fall into this category, including severe flexion distraction injuries and facet joint dislocations (Figures 7.12 and 7.13).

Further reading

Oakley P, Brohi K, Wilson A *et al.* Guidelines for initial management and assessment of spinal injury. British Trauma Society, 2002 *Injury* 2003; **34**: 405–425.

Van Goethem J, Maes M, Ozsarlak O *et al.* Imaging in spinal trauma. *European Radiology* 2005; **15**: 582–590.

Cassar-Pullicino VN & Imhof H. Spinal trauma – an imaging approach.

Wintermark M, Mouhsine E, Theumann N & Mordasini P. Thoracolumbar spine fractures in patients who have sustained severe trauma: depiction with multi-detector CT. *Radiology* 2003; **227**: 681–689.

CHAPTER 8

Vascular Trauma and Interventional Radiology

Clare L. Bent and Matthew B. Matson

The Royal London Hospital, London, UK

OVERVIEW

- A number of endovascular techniques are available to assist the surgeon in patients with haemorrhage following trauma
- Endovascular treatment with stent-grafts is emerging as the first-line treatment option for thoracic aortic injury
- In selected patients with abdominal solid organ injury, embolization can avoid the need for open surgery and reduced splenectomy and nephrectomy rates
- Embolization is preferable to open surgery as the first-line treatment for pelvic haemorrhage
- Covered stents can be used to restore flow and arrest haemorrhage from injured vessels

---

Box 8.1 **Types of embolic material**

- Soluble gelatine sponge
- Polyvinyl alcohol paricles
- Histoacryl glue
- Metal coils
- Vascular plugs

Introduction

Vascular injury, including arterial transection, intimal damage, dissection, pseudoaneurysm and arteriovenous fistula may result following blunt or penetrating trauma. In the majority, open surgical repair is the gold standard treatment option but may be challenging due to co-existent injuries, excessive bleeding, contaminated surgical fields and anatomical distortion.

Endovascular techniques are routinely used in the elective setting for a range of vascular diseases and this has led to their use in the trauma setting. Angiography allows rapid diagnosis of arterial injury with the option for immediate treatment with a variety of endovascular techniques, including balloon occlusion, stent-graft insertion and transcatheter embolization.

Endovascular techniques provide an opportunity to improve trauma care by serving as either a primary method of treatment or a temporary measure until definitive treatment can be instigated.

Interventional radiology techniques

Angiography

Computed tomography (CT) is commonly used to diagnose solid organ injury in trauma, and improvements in multidetector CT

(MDCT) design allow simultaneous assessment of vascular injury, leading to its increasing use in this setting. However, angiography remains the gold standard investigation for diagnosis of arterial injury, allowing prompt diagnosis of acute haemorrhage and definitive endovascular treatment in the same sitting.

Balloon occlusion

Inflation of an occlusion balloon proximal to a bleeding point can achieve rapid haemostasis, minimize blood loss at surgery and aid identification of a transected retracted artery during technically challenging surgical repair.

Stent insertion

Bare-metal stent insertion is often used for intimal tears or arterial dissection to restore flow in traumatized arteries.

Covered stents may be used in arterial rupture to stop bleeding by covering the breach in the vessel wall. They may also be used to exclude false aneurysms and seal arteriovenous fistulas, while maintaining flow in the artery.

Transcatheter embolization

Embolization is the selective delivery of thrombogenic material into a target vessel to cause intentional vessel occlusion with resultant haemostasis. A number of different embolic materials are available (Box 8.1), depending, for example, on the size of the target vessel and the need for a permanent or temporary result.

Type of vascular injury and interventional radiological techniques

Traumatic aortic injury (TAI)

Thoracic aortic rupture occurs in up to 20% of road traffic accident fatalities. On-scene survival is 2–5%. Of patients who survive a TAI,

---

ABC of Imaging in Trauma. By Leonard J. King and David C. Wherry
Published 2010 by Blackwell Publishing

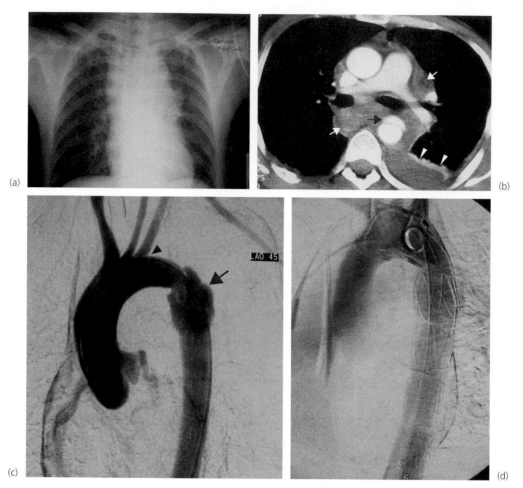

(a)　(b)　(c)　(d)

Figure 8.1 Traumatic aortic injury following a high-speed motor vehicle collision. (a) Chest radiograph demonstrates mediastinal widening. (b) Axial contrast-enhanced CT demonstrates a mediastinal haematoma (white arrows) extending into the left hemi-thorax (white arrowheads) and aortic injury with contrast outside the true lumen of the descending thoracic aorta (black arrow). (c) At aortography there is irregularity in the aortic contour (black arrow) 3 cm distal to the left subclavian artery (black arrowhead) confirming injury. (d) Subsequent aortography following stent placement demonstrates exclusion of the traumatic aortic injury (TAI).

the aortic isthmus is involved in 80–90% due to a posterior attachment by the ligamentum arteriosum. The majority occur following rapid deceleration (e.g. road traffic accidents), therefore patients frequently have concomitant injuries.

Management of TAI is challenging; strict blood pressure control is vital to prevent aortic rupture, but if head or spinal injuries are present, hypotension could potentially worsen neurological outcome.

Traditionally, treatment of TAI involved left thoracotomy, aortic cross-clamping, extracorporeal bypass and insertion of an interposition graft. However, such definitive surgery is associated with high morbidity and mortality, particularly in patients with severe co-existing injuries.

Endovascular treatment usually involves the placement of a single stent-graft from a common femoral approach into the injured aorta distal to the left subclavian artery (Figure 8.1). Because of the minimally invasive nature of this technique, many

specialists feel that thoracic aortic stent-graft insertion has become the first-line treatment option in this scenario.

Visceral injury

Solid abdominal organ injuries can occur following blunt or penetrating trauma. Patients with evidence of visceral injury, such as intra-abdominal fluid seen on focused ultrasound, and who are unstable, require emergency surgery. Stable patients, however, are often further assessed with CT, enabling accurate diagnosis of organ injury and localization of haemorrhage. In this group of patients, those with evidence of localized bleeding on CT or those with clinical evidence of continued bleeding can be considered for endovascular therapy.

Splenic trauma

The spleen is the commonest solid abdominal organ to be injured. Transcatheter embolization is used as an alternative to open

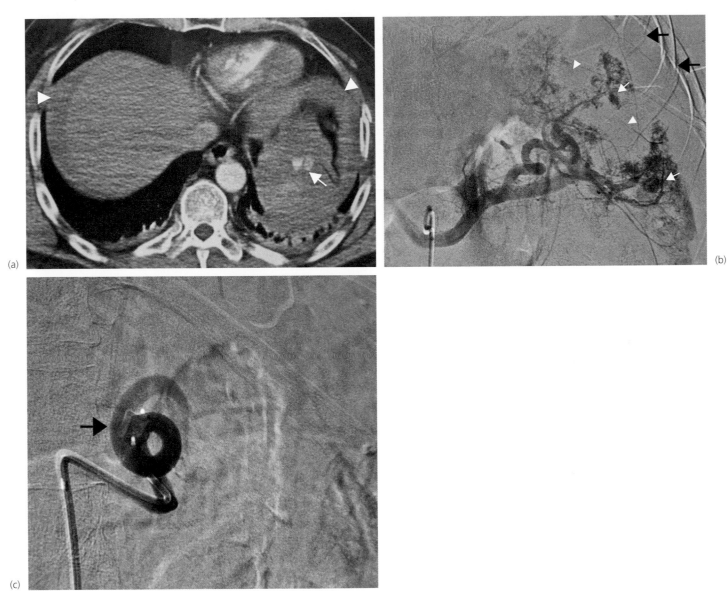

Figure 8.2 Traumatic splenic injury. (a) Axial contrast-enhanced CT demonstrates left-sided rib fractures, free intra-abdominal fluid (white arrowheads) and contrast extravasation in the spleen (white arrow) consistent with active bleeding. (b) Angiography via a catheter placed at the coeliac axis origin shows areas of avascularity due to splenic laceration (white arrowheads) and contrast blushing indicating acute bleeding (white arrows). The rib fractures are also shown (black arrows). (c) Subsequent selective splenic artery angiography following nitinol vascular plug deployment (black arrow) demonstrates thrombosis of the splenic artery and haemostasis.

surgery, aiming to achieve haemostasis with organ preservation, minimizing the risk of overwhelming sepsis that may occur following splenectomy.

Embolization of the splenic artery is performed via a common femoral artery approach. The most common technique involves placement of metallic coils via a catheter into the splenic artery just distal to the dorsal pancreatic artery (Figure 8.2). This reduces splenic blood flow and arterial pressure while preserving collateral flow, thus maintaining the viability of the spleen.

Non-operative management of splenic injury is successful even in cases of high-grade trauma, with reported salvage rates of up to 84%. Complications of this technique are rare but include non-target embolization, splenic infarction or abscess formation, and splenic artery dissection.

Hepatic trauma

Liver lacerations and bleeding following trauma are often clearly delineated on CT imaging (Figure 8.3a). In the majority, bleeding originates from the hepatic artery and it is therefore important to assess portal vein patency when planning management strategies. The combination of poor surgical results (mortality >50%) and a high incidence of spontaneous resolution of haemorrhage has led

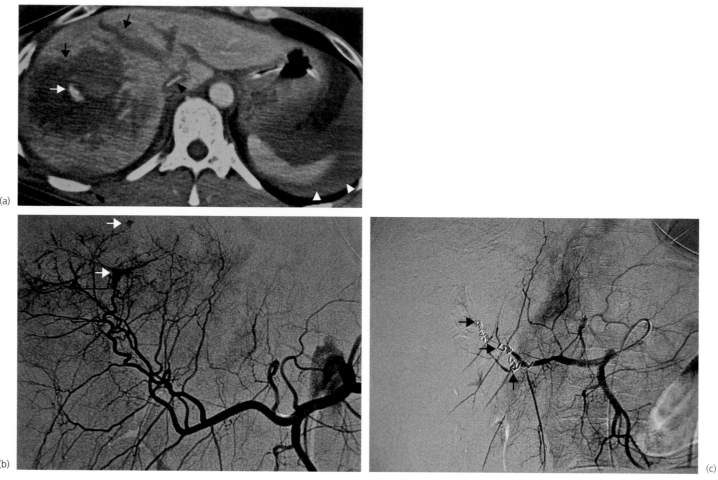

(a)

(b)

(c)

Figure 8.3 Hepatic injury following blunt trauma. (a) Axial contrast-enhanced CT demonstrates free fluid (white arrowheads), areas of low density representing hepatic contusions (black arrows) and extravasation of contrast within the right lobe of the liver (white arrow). The IVC is also flattened due to hypovolaemia (black arrowhead). (b) Selective hepatic artery angiography demonstrates two areas of contrast blushing consistent with acute bleeding (white arrows). (c) Repeat angiography following selective catheter placement and embolization with platinum coils (black arrows) demonstrates vessel occlusion and haemostasis.

to a shift towards non-operative management in hepatic trauma. If CT imaging demonstrates active extravasation of contrast or hepatic injury with continued hypotension, angiography is indicated (Figure 8.3b).

Angiography of the liver allows localization of bleeding, pseudoaneurysm or arteriovenous fistulae, followed by selective embolization of the abnormality (Figure 8.3c). Super-selective techniques with gelatine sponge, coils or micro-coils can achieve haemostasis while maintaining the majority of hepatic artery flow with low complication rates. Portal vein occlusion is a contraindication to hepatic artery embolization in this scenario.

Hepatic artery embolization is preferential to surgery due to reported technical success rates of 90%. Even in complex and penetrating hepatic injuries, survival rates following embolization are high.

Renal trauma

The kidney is the most commonly injured retroperitoneal structure following blunt and penetrating trauma. Because of its retroperi-

toneal location, surgical exploration can be challenging, particularly in the presence of large retroperitoneal haematomas, which can hinder local haemostatic techniques. As a consequence, the majority of renal injuries are now treated using conservative or endovascular management strategies.

When there is evidence of renal haemorrhage on CT (Figure 8.4a), angiography commonly identifies a single bleeding point or pseudoaneurysm, allowing super-selective transcatheter embolization to obtain haemostasis while minimizing tissue loss (Figures 8.4b & 8.4c). Embolization with soluble gelatine sponge is preferable to coil placement because it has greater potential for subsequent re-vascularization.

Pelvic injury

Pelvic haemorrhage secondary to trauma can originate from arterial, venous or osseous sources. Traditionally, patients with significant pelvic ring fractures (Figure 8.5a) undergo immediate external fixation to reduce the fracture or dislocation and decrease the pelvic space, thus aiding the tamponade effect. However, contin-

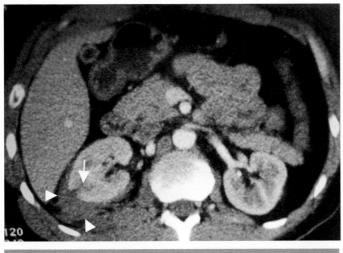

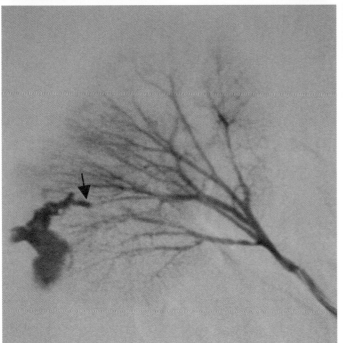

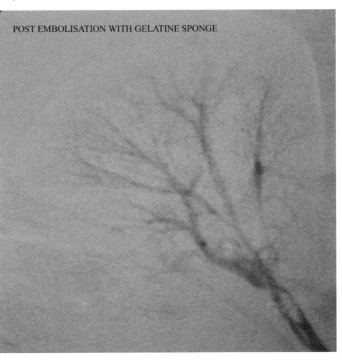

POST EMBOLISATION WITH GELATINE SPONGE

Figure 8.4 Renal injury following blunt trauma to the right flank. (a) Axial contrast-enhanced CT indicates a renal laceration (white arrow) with adjacent peri-nephric haematoma (white arrowheads). (b) Initial renal angiography shows acute extravasation of contrast (black arrow) from a mid- to lower-pole arcuate artery. (c) Repeat angiography following embolization with gelatine sponge demonstrates haemostasis.

ued haemorrhage may indicate arterial damage necessitating intervention.

Open surgery for pelvic haemorrhage has a reported mortality rate of 40%, and frequently the source of bleeding is not positively identified. Many believe disruption of fascial planes during surgical exploration reduces the tamponade effect on the pelvic haematoma, increasing the risk of blood loss.

Only around 5% of patients with pelvic trauma require angiographic assessment. Angiography and embolization of an unstable patient with pelvic trauma within three hours of presentation has been shown to reduce mortality. Of the patients requiring embolization, vertical shear fractures represent the commonest underlying traumatic abnormality (52%).

Pelvic angiography is performed via a common femoral approach (Figure 8.5b). A catheter is passed into each internal iliac artery and contrast administered to look for extravasation, which is present in approximately 50% of cases. If evidence of bleeding is seen then embolization is required, and soluble gelatine sponge is routinely used (Figure 8.5c). Empirical embolization of the internal iliac arteries can be performed if no bleeding is identified on angiography, but CT or clinical evidence of haemorrhage exists. Despite technical success rates ranging from 85 to 100%, mortality remains high at 43%, due to concomitant injuries.

Complications following pelvic embolization are rare. Non-target embolization is avoided by stable catheter position. Choice of embolic agent is important to prevent distal embolization, which

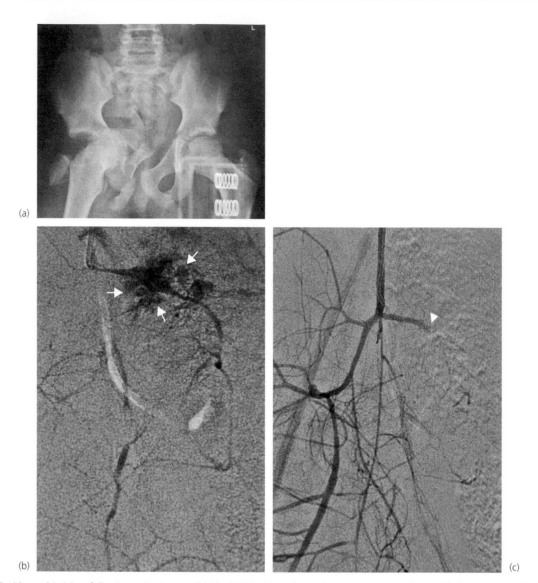

Figure 8.5 Child with a pelvic injury following major trauma. (a) The initial plain radiograph demonstrates multiple pelvic fractures. A pelvic brace is in situ. (b) Subsequent right internal iliac artery angiography shows contrast extravasation consistent with acute bleeding (white arrows). (c) Repeat angiography following embolization with gelatine sponge (white arrowhead) demonstrates successful haemostasis.

may lead to tissue necrosis. Bilateral internal iliac artery embolization can lead to impotence in male patients, therefore neurological injuries should be recorded prior to the procedure.

On completion, non-selective angiography of the pelvis is performed to exclude other sites of extravasation or collateral vessels causing retrograde haemorrhage requiring further embolization.

Arterial injury involving larger calibre vessels (e.g. common iliac or external iliac artery) can be managed with endovascular stent insertion (Figure 8.6). Bare-metal and covered stents are available in a variety of diameters and lengths, dependent on extent of injury.

In catastrophic haemorrhage, an aortic occlusion balloon placed within the distal aorta can often be a life-saving manoeuvre to aid resuscitation until definitive treatment can be instigated.

Peripheral vascular injury

Extremity arterial injury most frequently occurs as a result of penetrating trauma, either from a stabbing or indirectly by fracture fragments. CT can depict both bony trauma and allow identification of active extravasation of contrast from bleeding arteries.

Expeditious treatment is required to prevent life-threatening exsanguination and to ensure limb salvage. Surgical management remains the gold standard; however, arterial haemorrhage requires proximal and distal control, sometimes necessitating long and complex surgical approaches. In addition, surgical repair following vascular trauma has been reported to have a 10–30% major complication rate and a 2% post-perioperative death rate.

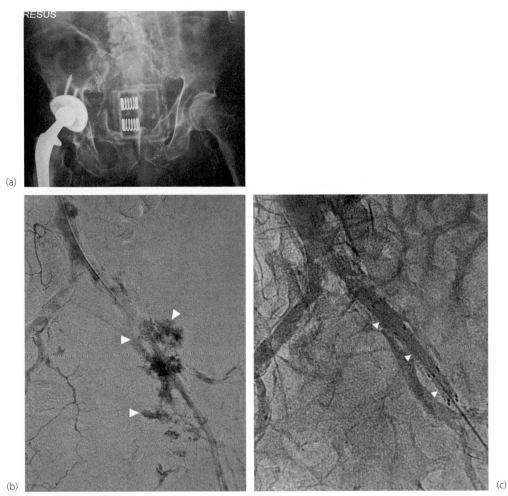

Figure 8.6 Adult patient with pelvic trauma from a motor vehicle collision. (a) The pelvic radiograph demonstrates a pelvic brace is in situ, previous right total hip replacement and multiple fractures. (b) Non-selective angiography shows extensive contrast extravasation in the region of the left external iliac artery (white arrowheads) due to rupture. (c) Repeat angiography following placement of two covered stent-grafts demonstrates haemostasis and restoration of arterial flow (white arrowheads).

Diagnosis of extremity vascular injury can be difficult, with absence of clinical signs in more than 20% of patients at presentation. Balloon occlusion proximal to the bleeding vessel offers rapid control of massive haemorrhage, aids resuscitation and minimizes blood loss during surgery.

Balloon inflation may also be of use during technically challenging vascular repair. A transected artery frequently retracts, requiring extensive surgical exploration to identify vessel stumps and allow re-anastomosis to restore continuity. Balloon inflation in this scenario may aid the identification process.

Endovascular stent insertion has been described for intimal injury and arterial dissection (Figure 8.7). Reports of bare-metal stent placement in the aorto-iliac, subclavian and carotid arteries are more common than lower extremity arteries; however, these are not adequate for management of a complete vessel wall injury,

which requires placement of a covered stent. Published data on the role of stent-graft placement following extremity vascular trauma shows great promise. Despite concerns regarding long-term complications and durability, short- and mid-term results have been extremely good.

Transcatheter arterial embolization following extremity vascular trauma is well described, particularly in the profunda femoris and tibial arteries (Figure 8.8). Where arterial injury involves a vessel with an existing collateral circulation, distal and proximal embolization should be performed to prevent retrograde haemorrhage. Fractures of the tibia and fibula frequently cause arterial injury, with consequent compartment syndrome from acute haemorrhage. In this scenario, as long as one tibial vessel is intact, embolization can be performed until haemostasis is achieved.

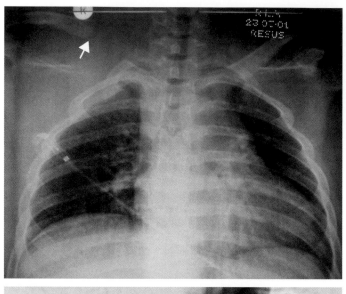

(a)

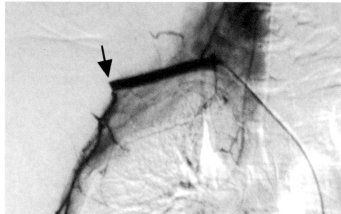

(b)

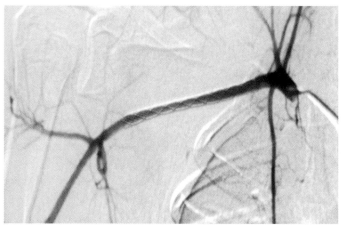

(c)

Figure 8.7 Adult patient with blunt trauma to the upper thorax and an ischaemic right upper limb. (a) The initial chest radiograph shows a displaced fracture of the right clavicle (white arrow) and associated soft tissue swelling. (b) Selective angiography of the right subclavian artery demonstrates abrupt cessation of contrast flow (black arrow) indicating arterial injury. A wire was subsequently passed into the distal segment and a covered stent deployed. (c) Repeat angiography confirms restoration of blood flow to the right upper limb.

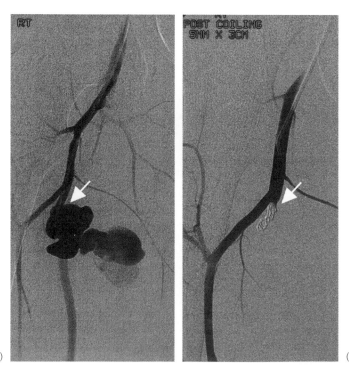

(a)

(b)

Figure 8.8 Adult patient with a stab wound to the right thigh. (a) Selective right profunda artery angiography demonstrates arterial bleeding from a branch of the profunda femoris artery. (b) Repeat angiography following coil embolization (white arrows) demonstrates haemostasis.

Further reading

Dyet JF, Ettles DF, Nicholson AA & Wilson SE. *Textbook of Endovascular Procedures*. Churchill Livingstone, Oxford, 2000.

Kessel D & Robertson I. *Interventional Radiology: a survival guide*, 2nd edn. Churchill Livingstone, Oxford, 2005.

Nicholson AA. Vascular radiology in trauma. *Cardiovascular and Interventional Radiology* 2004; **27**: 105–120.

Reuben BC, Whitten MG, Sarfati M & Kraiss LW. Increasing use of endovascular therapy in acute arterial injuries: analysis of the National Trauma Data Bank. *Journal of Vascular Surgery* 2007; **46**: 1222–1226.

Sclafani SJA, Schaftan GW & Scalea TM. Non-operative salvage of computed tomography diagnosed splenic injuries: utilisation of angiography for triage and embolisation for haemostasis. *Journal of Trauma Injury, Infection and Critical Care* 1995; **39**: 818–827.

CHAPTER 9

Upper Limb Injuries

James Teh[1], David Gay[1] and Richard A. Schaefer[2]

[1]Nuffield Orthopaedic Centre, Oxford, Oxfordshire, UK
[2]Uniformed Services University of the Health Sciences, Bethesda, MD, USA

OVERVIEW

- More than 80% of scapular fractures are associated with injuries of the chest, head or spine
- Scapulothoracic dissociation often results in neurovascular injury
- Anterior dislocations account for more than 95% of shoulder dislocations
- Posterior dislocations often occur as a result of severe muscle spasms associated with electric shocks or fits
- In children, the avulsed medial epicondyle ossification centre may be mistaken for the trochlear ossification centre
- Forearm fractures are often associated with dislocations of the elbow or wrist
- Carpal dislocations are described in relation to the lunate

Introduction

The initial management of major trauma should always focus on the greatest threat to life first. Only when patients have been stabilized should specific imaging of upper limb trauma be considered. Major injuries to the upper limb can be evaluated using the ABCS principle (Box 9.1).

Imaging of major upper limb trauma utilizes radiography, computed tomography (CT), magnetic resonance imaging (MRI) and ultrasound. Most decisions regarding the management of major upper limb trauma can be made using plain radiographs and CT. Radiographs are invariably the initial investigation and should be obtained in at least two orthogonal planes. CT, with its excellent spatial resolution and multiplanar capability, is useful for demonstrating fractures when conventional radiography is inconclusive. CT is also essential in the delineation of complex fractures and has a key role in surgical planning, particularly when two- and three-dimensional reformats are utilized. CT angiography also allows evaluation of associated vascular injuries.

Shoulder girdle injuries

The shoulder girdle consists of the humerus, scapula and clavicle.

ABC of Imaging in Trauma. By Leonard J. King and David C. Wherry
Published 2010 by Blackwell Publishing

Box 9.1 **ABCS of assessment of plain radiographs**

A Adequacy
A Alignment
B Bones
C Cartilage and joints
S Soft tissues

ABCS of assessment
Adequacy

At least two radiographs in orthogonal planes should be obtained. The anteroposterior (AP) view is obtained with the arm externally rotated and the greater tuberosity in profile. The second radiograph can be an axial view, a "Y" view or a modified axial view. On the axial view the humeral head should sit on the glenoid like a golf ball on a tee. On the "Y" view the humeral head should be projected over the centre of the glenoid.

Alignment

Glenohumeral joint: the joint space should be even and the humeral head congruent with the glenoid.

Acromioclavicular joint: the inferior margin of clavicle should align with the inferior margin of acromion on the AP view, although slight variation may be present in up to 20% of asymptomatic individuals.

Bones

The cortical margin of each bone should be smooth with no breaks or buckles. Impacted fractures may look sclerotic. The trabecular pattern should appear continuous. The ribs should also be examined.

Cartilage and joint

The glenohumeral joint space should be congruent. Loss of joint space may occur due to cartilage loss or technical factors. The normal acromioclavicular joint distance is less than 7 mm and the coracoclavicular distance is normally less than 14 mm.

Soft tissues

The glenohumeral joint should be assessed for a fat–fluid level indicating a lipohaemarthrosis due to an intra-articular fracture.

Acromioclavicular joint disruption may result in soft tissue swelling. Surgical emphysema and pneumothorax should also be looked for.

Scapular fractures

Scapular fractures are uncommon, accounting for 1% of all fractures and around 5% of shoulder girdle injuries. They are usually the result of high-energy impact due to falls and road traffic accidents. In more than 80% of patients there are associated injuries to the chest, head or spine, which may be life threatening (Box 9.2).

Around 50% of fractures involve the scapular body or spine, 25% the neck and 10% the acromion or coracoid (Figure 9.1). Scapular fractures are often first detected on chest radiographs obtained as part of the primary survey. If a fracture is seen or suspected, dedicated shoulder radiographs should be obtained. CT is usually required for further delineation of the fracture and to evaluate associated thoracic injuries. Most scapular fractures can be managed conservatively; however, special attention should be paid to significantly displaced fractures of the glenoid cavity or neck, and double disruptions of the superior shoulder suspensory complex (SSSC) as these may require surgery.

The classification of scapular fractures involving the glenoid cavity is shown in Box 9.3. Fractures displaced by more than 10 mm or involving more than 25% of the cavity should be considered unstable (Figure 9.2).

The superior shoulder suspensory complex is a bone and soft-tissue ring secured to the trunk by a superior strut (middle third of the clavicle) and inferior strut (lateral scapular body and spine) from which the upper extremity is suspended. The ring is composed of the glenoid, coracoid process, coracoclavicular ligament, distal clavicle, acromioclavicular joint and acromion.

Traumatic disruptions of a solitary component of the SSSC are common (e.g. simple clavicle fracture). With sufficient force, the ring may fail in two or more places (double disruption), leading to altered shoulder biomechanics and instability. If there is significant displacement (>1 cm) or instability, surgical reduction may be indicated.

The floating shoulder is an uncommon but important injury consisting of ipsilateral fractures of the clavicle and scapular neck (Figure 9.3). Ligament disruption associated with isolated scapular neck fractures may result in the functional equivalent of this injury.

Scapulothoracic dissociation is a rare and potentially fatal injury. The scapula is distracted from the body and is the equivalent of a closed forequarter amputation. Associated rib injury is common and there is often neurovascular injury necessitating angiography. Plain radiographs demonstrate lateral displacement of the scapula with massive soft tissue swelling and a clavicle

---

Box 9.2 **Frequency of injuries associated with scapular fractures**

Rib fractures	Up to 45%
Pulmonary injury	Up to 55%
Humerus fractures	12%
Brachial plexus injury	10%
Skull fractures	25%
Major vascular injury	11%
Splenic injury requiring splenectomy	8%

Box 9.3 **Classification of fractures involving the glenoid cavity**

Type I	Rim fracture
Type II	Glenoid fossa fracture exiting at lateral border of the scapula
Type III	Glenoid fossa fracture exiting at superior border of the scapula
Type IV	Glenoid fossa fracture exiting at the medial border of the scapula
Type V	Glenoid fossa fracture exiting at two or more borders of the scapula
Type VI	Comminuted fracture

TYPES OF SCAPULA FRACTURES

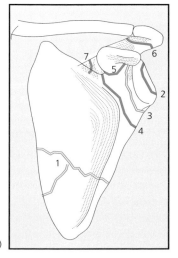

1. Body

2. Glenoid rim or articular surface

3. Anatomic neck

4. Surgical neck

5. Coracoid process

6. Acromion process

7. Spine

(a)

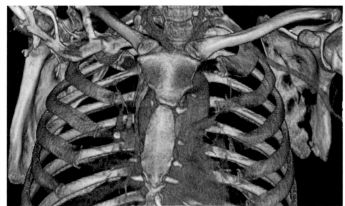

(b)

Figure 9.1 (a) Diagram illustrating the anatomical types of scapular fractures. (b) Three-dimensional volume-rendered CT image of a scapular body fracture.

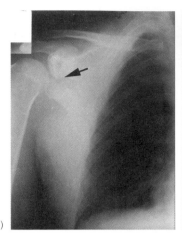

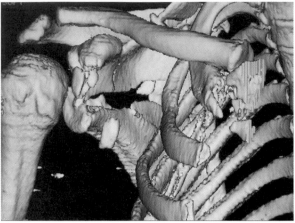

(a)

(b)

Figure 9.2 2 Glenoid cavity fracture. (a) AP radiograph showing a displaced glenoid cavity (TypeV) fracture (arrow). (b) Surface rendered three-dimensional CT reformat showing the position of the fracture fragments.

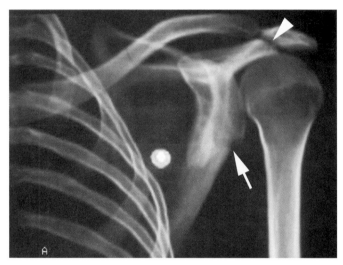

Figure 9.3 Floating shoulder. Transparent three-dimensional CT reformat shows fractures of the scapular neck (arrow) and acromion (arrowhead), indicating a double disruption of the superior shoulder suspensory complex.

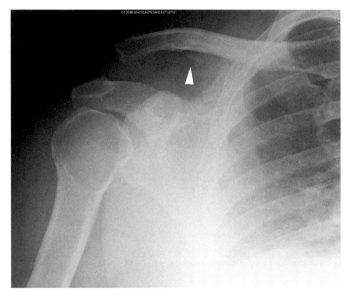

Figure 9.5 Acromioclavicular joint (ACJ) dislocation (Type 3). Loss of ACJ alignment with avulsion of the clavicular attachment of the coracoclavicular ligament (arrowhead).

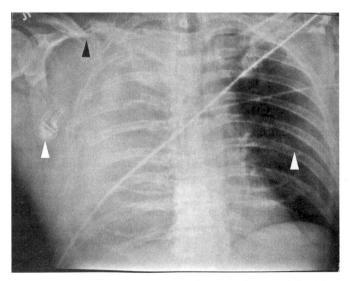

Figure 9.4 Scapulo-thoracic dissociation. There is a white-out of the right hemithorax, indicating a large haemothorax. The right scapula is laterally displaced (white arrowheads indicate the position of the inferior tips of the scapulae). There is a fracture of the right clavicle (black arrowhead) and multiple rib fractures.

fracture or acromioclavicular joint separation. On a well-centred chest radiograph the distance from the midline of the spine to the tips of both scapulae is unequal (Figure 9.4).

Clavicle fractures

Fractures of the clavicle are common and normally due to a direct blow or a fall on to an outstretched hand. Approximately 80% of clavicle fractures occur in the middle third, with inferior displacement of the distal fragment. Around 15% involve the lateral third and 5% involve the medial third. Posterior fracture displacement can occasionally result in injury to the subclavian vessels or brachial plexus.

Acromioclavicular joint (ACJ) injury

Acromioclavicular joint injuries are common in young adults, occurring after falls on to the shoulder or outstretched hand (Figure 9.5). Injuries are graded according to the Rockwood classification system (Figure 9.6).

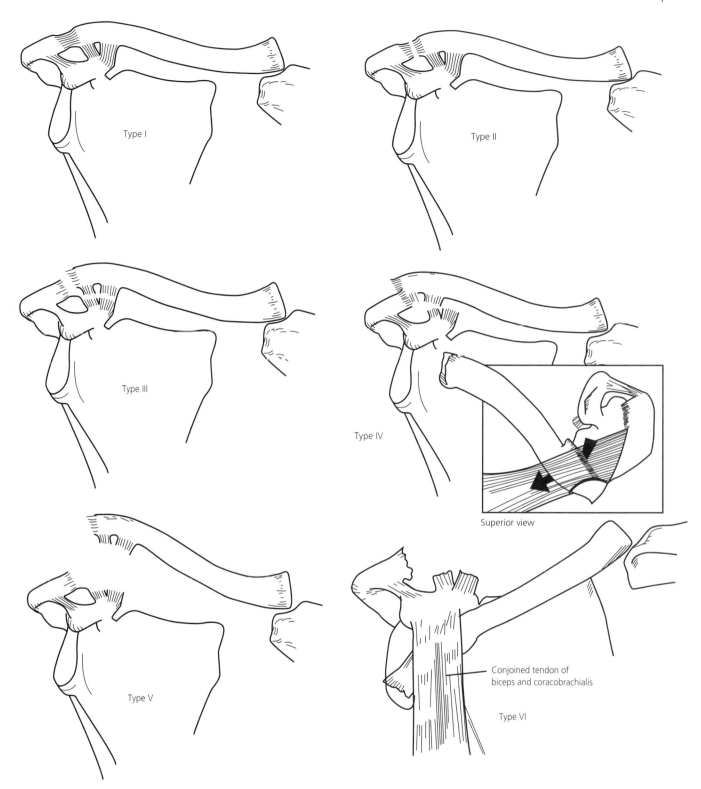

Figure 9.6 Rockwood classification of ACJ injury

I   Minor ligament injury, normal plain radiograph
II   Widening of ACJ, normal coracoclavicular distance
III Widening of ACJ and coracoclavicular distance
IV   Posterior dislocation, with button holing of clavicle through trapezius
V   Severe upward displacement of clavicle
VI   Inferior displacement of clavicle

Sternoclavicular joint injury

Dislocation of the sternoclavicular joint is an uncommon injury that may be difficult to detect radiographically due to overlying structures, and CT is recommended for confirmation and delineation. Most dislocations are anterosuperior (Figure 9.7). Posterosuperior dislocation is less common but may be associated with damage to mediastinal structures.

Shoulder dislocation
Anterior dislocation

The shoulder is the most frequently dislocated joint, accounting for around 50% of all dislocations. Ninety-five percent of shoulder dislocations are anterior. Plain radiographs in two orthogonal

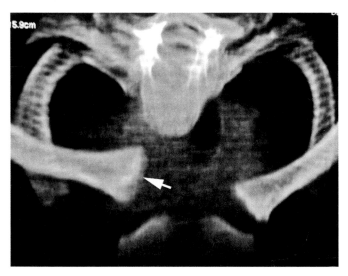

Figure 9.7 Superior dislocation of the sternoclavicular joint. Three-dimensional CT reformat showing superior dislocation of the clavicle (arrow).

planes should be performed to confirm the injury and identify associated fractures. On AP radiographs the glenohumeral joint loses congruity with inferomedial displacement of the humeral head. On the axial view or the "Y" view the humeral head lies anterior to the glenoid (Figure 9.8). These dislocations can be classified according to the position of the humeral head, which may lie subclavicular, subcoracoid, subglenoid or intrathoracic (Figure 9.9).

Complications of shoulder dislocation are common. In up to 50% of patients, indentation of the posterolateral humeral head by the glenoid results in a hatchet shaped "Hill Sachs" impaction fracture. In around 15% of cases there is a fracture of the greater tuberosity, and a Bankhart fracture of the anterior–inferior margin of the glenoid occurs in up to 10% of patients. Soft tissue or capsulolabral injuries cannot be demonstrated on plain radiographs. Patients with these injuries usually present with chronic pain and shoulder instability, which is best evaluated by MR arthrography. Associated rotator cuff tears tend to occur in older patients.

Posterior dislocation

Posterior dislocation (Box 9.4) can result from trauma but usually occurs as a result of severe muscle contractions due an epileptic fit or electric shock. The humeral head is forced posteriorly in internal rotation, resulting in a light bulb appearance of the humeral head on AP radiographs. AP radiographs also demonstrate increased distance (>6 mm) between the anterior rim of the glenoid fossa and the medial aspect of the humeral head, and may reveal two nearly parallel lines in the superomedial aspect of the humeral head. The more medial line is the subchondral bone of the humeral head, and the more lateral "trough line" represents the margin of a trough-like compression fracture due to impaction of the anterior aspect of the humeral head against the posterior glenoid rim (Figures 9.10 and 9.11).

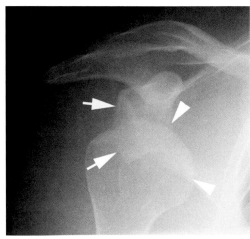
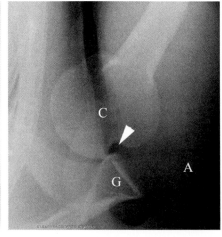

(a)   (b)

Figure 9.8 Anterior shoulder dislocation. (a) AP radiograph demonstrates subcoracoid anterior dislocation. The glenoid fossa (arrows) sits empty with inferior displacement of the humeral head (arrowhead). (b) Modified axial view demonstrates the position of the acromion (A), glenoid (G) and coracoid (C), with the humeral head lying anteriorly, projected over the coracoid. There is a Hill-Sachs deformity (arrowhead).

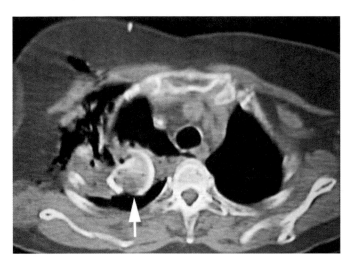

Figure 9.9 Intra-thoracic shoulder dislocation. The arrow points to the humeral head.

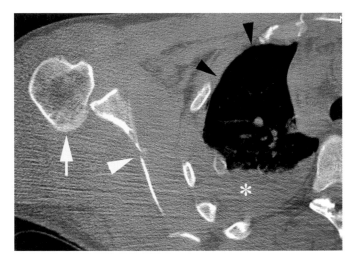

Figure 9.11 Posterior dislocation on CT. The humeral head lies posteriorly (arrow). There is an associated scapular fracture, a pneumothorax (black arrows) and a haemothorax (asterisk).

Box 9.4 **Radiographic signs of posterior dislocation**

- Light bulb appearance of humeral head
- Trough line of humeral head
- Rim sign = increased distance (>6mm) between anterior rim of glenoid fossa and medial aspect of humeral head.

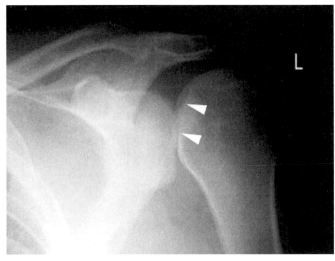

Figure 9.10 Posterior dislocation. The AP view shows a light bulb appearance of the humeral head with a trough line (arrowheads).

Proximal humerus injuries

Fractures of the head and neck of humerus are common in the elderly, usually occurring after a fall. Plain films will usually demonstrate the injury, but CT is often required for surgical planning. There may be associated neurovascular injury, particularly involving the radial nerve.

The proximal humerus can be divided into four parts: the articular surface, greater tuberosity, lesser tuberosity and humeral shaft.

Using the modified Neer classification (Figure 9.12) fractures are divided into the number of parts according to the degree of displacement of the fracture fragments by more than 1 cm, or angulation between fracture fragments of over 45 degrees. More than 80% of fractures are one-part, while four-part fractures comprise less than 5% of cases. Most fractures are minimally displaced and treated non-operatively. Three- and four-part fractures often require surgical management (Figure 9.13).

Elbow region injury

The elbow is a complex joint both anatomically and functionally, comprising of three articulations.

ABCS of assessment
Adequacy
AP and lateral radiographs should be obtained.

Alignment
Two lines should be drawn to exclude dislocation. The radio-capitellar line is drawn along the mid-shaft of the radius and should intersect the capitellum. The anterior humeral line is drawn down the anterior humeral cortex and should intersect the middle third of the capitellum.

Bones
The coronoid and olecranon fossae give the appearance of an hour-glass, in which there should be no cortical breaks.

In children, ossification centres around the elbow must be recognized. These appear in a set order: CRITOL.

    Capitellum
    Radial head
    Internal (medial) epicondyle
    Trochlea
    Olecranon
    Lateral epicondyle

FOUR-SEGMENT CLASSIFICATION OF FRACTURES OF THE PPROXIMAL HUMERUS

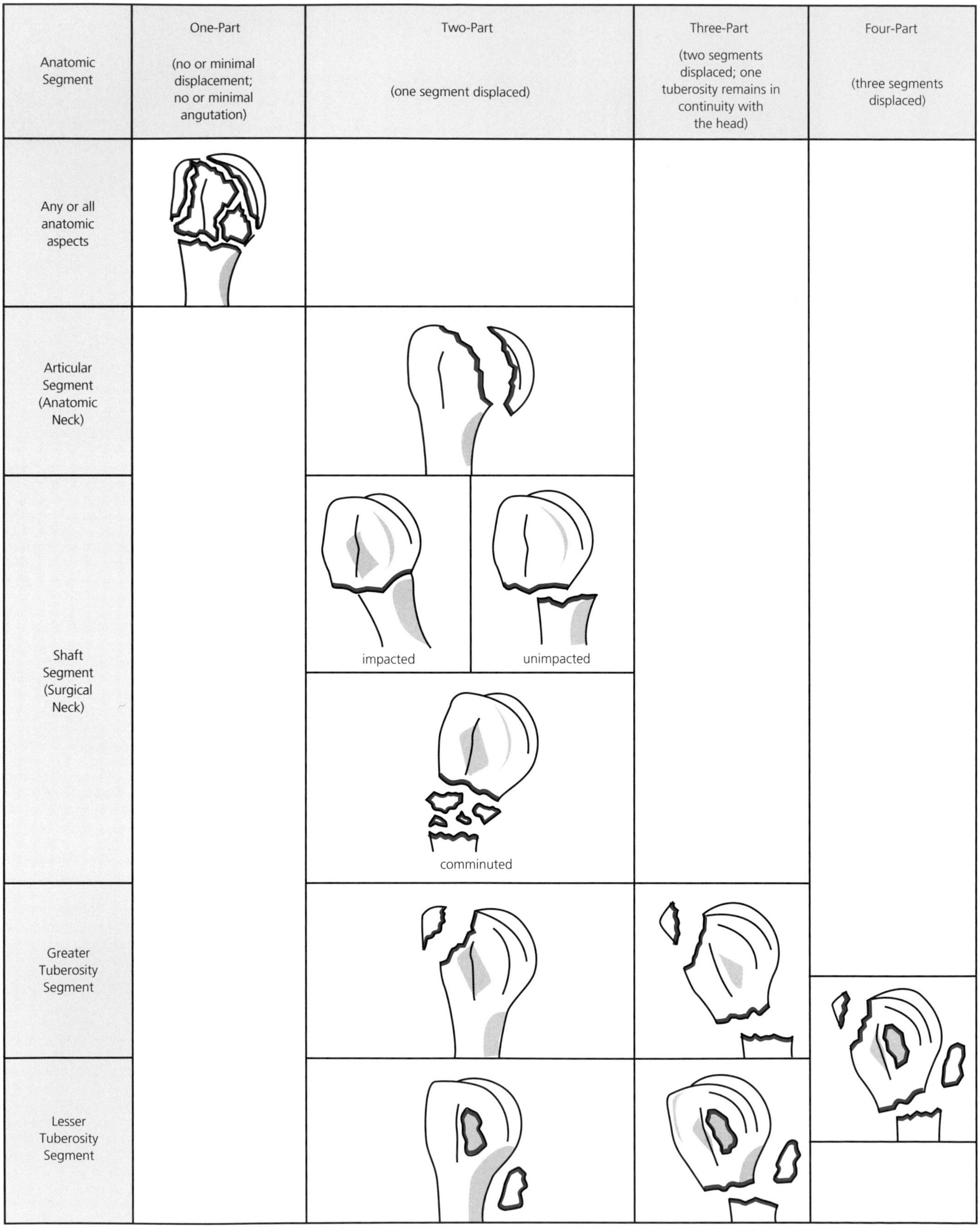

Anatomic Segment	One-Part (no or minimal displacement; no or minimal angutation)	Two-Part (one segment displaced)		Three-Part (two segments displaced; one tuberosity remains in continuity with the head)	Four-Part (three segments displaced)
Any or all anatomic aspects					
Articular Segment (Anatomic Neck)					
Shaft Segment (Surgical Neck)		impacted	unimpacted		
		comminuted			
Greater Tuberosity Segment					
Lesser Tuberosity Segment					

Figure 9.12 Neer classification of proximal humeral fractures.

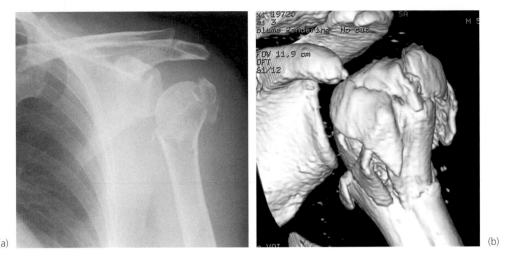

(a)   (b)

Figure 9.13 Three-part fracture of the humerus. (a) AP radiograph showing displaced fractures of the greater and lesser tuberosities and the surgical neck of the humerus. (b) Three-dimensional CT reformat showing the position of the fracture fragments.

The internal epicondyle always appears before the trochlea: "I before T". If the trochlear ossification centre looks as if it is present, but the medial epicondyle ossification centre is not seen, an avulsed medial epicondyle should be suspected as the cause of this appearance.

Cartilage and joints

The forearm bones, along with the proximal and distal radio-ulnar joints can be considered as a ring. Therefore, if a fracture is seen in one part of the ring, a further injury in the remainder of the ring should be sought.

Soft tissues

The anterior fat pad lies in the coronoid fossa and is normally seen adjacent to the humerus as a well-defined lucency. An effusion or haemarthrosis displaces the anterior fat pad, giving the sail sign. The posterior fat pad lies in the olecranon fossa. where is not normally seen and if visible indicates that an effusion is present.

Fractures around the elbow occur either as a result of direct impact or a fall on to the outstretched hand. The pattern of injury is highly dependent on patient age. In children, supracondylar fractures predominate, while in adults, radial head fractures tend to occur.

Distal humerus fractures

Fractures of the distal humerus are intra or extra-articular, and may be supracondylar, intercondylar or transcondylar (Figure 9.14). Isolated fractures of the epicondyles, capitellum or trochlea may also occur. The number of fracture fragments, the degree of depression of articular surfaces and the presence of loose bodies should be assessed.

Radiocapitellar dislocations are common in young children – usually sustained in the context of a pulled elbow rather than major trauma. The radiocapitellar line is disrupted.

Box 9.5 Mason classification of radial head fractures

Type 1	Undisplaced
Type 2	Marginal fractures with displacement
Type 3	Comminuted involving the entire radial head
Type 4	Fracture-dislocation

Radial head fractures

Radial head fractures may be classified according to the Mason classification (Box 9.5). The degree of involvement of the articular surface can be better assessed on CT (Figure 9.15).

Elbow dislocations

Elbow dislocations may be simple or complex. Simple dislocations are soft tissue injuries, classified by the direction of radial or ulnar displacement in relation to the distal part of the humerus. Posterior and posterolateral dislocations are the most common pattern, accounting for up to 90% of dislocations. If an elbow dislocation is present, AP and lateral radiographs of the entire forearm must be obtained to exclude an associated fracture.

Complex elbow dislocations are associated with fractures and/or neurovascular injuries. Coronoid process fractures occur in 10–15% of elbow dislocations and isolated fractures without dislocation are rare (Figure 9.16). Avulsion of the medial epicondyle may occur in association with elbow dislocation in children and may be mistaken for the trochlear ossification centre (Figure 9.17).

Forearm fracture-dislocations

The radius and ulna are attached by a strong interosseous ligament. If a displaced or angulated fracture occurs to one of these bones, the other is also usually fractured or there is dislocation of the proximal or distal radio-ulnar joints. A Monteggia fracture-dislocation is an ulnar fracture with a proximal radio-ulnar dislocation (Figure 9.18), usually resulting from a direct blow to the

FRACTURES OF THE DISTAL HUMERUS

Extra-articular—Epicondylar, Supracondylar

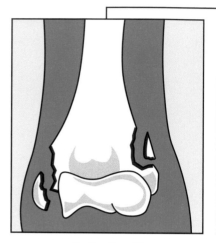

avulsion of medial
and/or lateral epicondyle

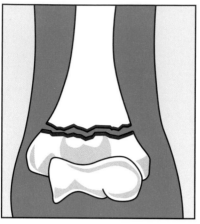

simple supracondylar fracture

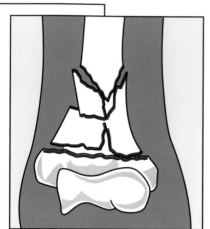

comminuted
supracondylar fracture

Intra-articular—Transcondylar

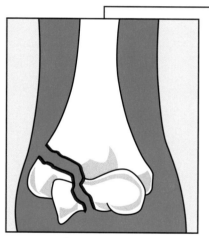

fracture of trochlea

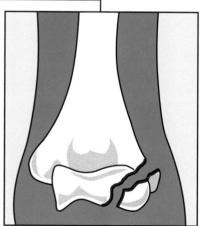

fracture of capitellum

Intra-articular—Bicondylar, Intercondylar

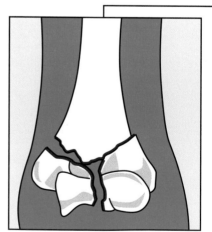

Y-shaped bicondylar fracture

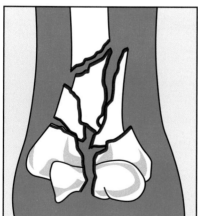

Y-shaped intercondylar fracture
with supracondylar comminution

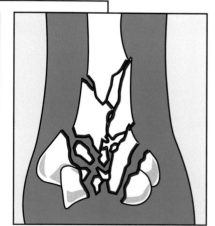

complex comminuted fracture

Figure 9.14 Diagram illustrating the Müller classification of distal humeral fractures.

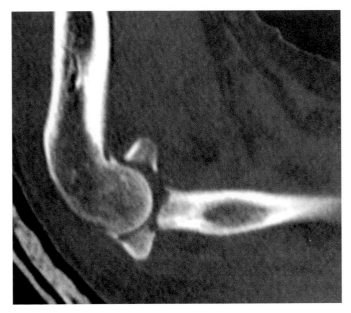

Figure 9.15 Sagittal reformatted CT image demonstrating a comminuted fracture of the radial head.

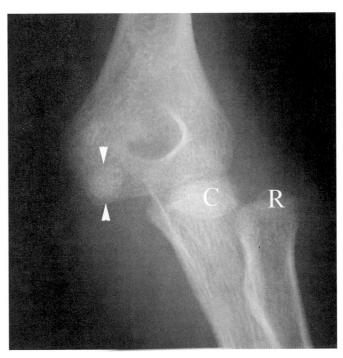

Figure 9.17 Posterior dislocation of the elbow with medial epicondyle avulsion in a child. The medial epicondyle ossification centre (arrowheads) could be mistaken for the trochlear ossification centre. The radius (R) and capitellum (C) are malaligned.

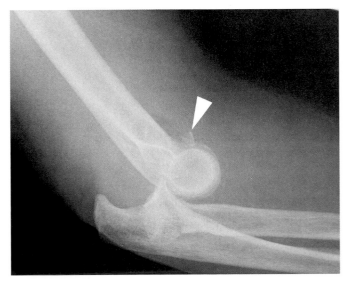

Figure 9.16 Complex posterior dislocation of the elbow. There is a posterior dislocation with a displaced fracture of the coronoid process (arrowhead).

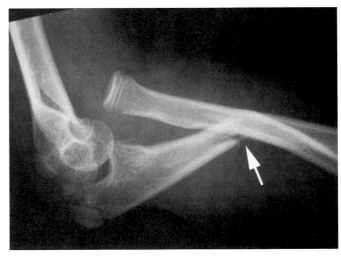

Figure 9.18 Monteggia fracture-dislocation in a child. The ulna is fractured (arrow) and there is dislocation of the proximal radioulnar and radiocapitellar joints.

posterior aspect of the ulna or forced pronation of the forearm during a fall.

A Galeazzi fracture-dislocation is a radial shaft fracture with a distal radio-ulnar joint dislocation. The Essex-Lopresti fracture-dislocation consists of a comminuted radial head fracture, a tear of the interosseous membrane and a distal radio-ulnar joint dislocation.

Wrist injury

ABCS of assessment
Adequacy
AP and lateral views should be centred over the joint. On the lateral view the radius and ulna should be superimposed. Suspected scaphoid fractures may require additional views.

Alignment
The carpal bones are divided into two rows, along which smooth curving lines can be drawn. The proximal carpal row comprises the scaphoid, lunate, triquetrum and pisiform. The distal row comprises the trapezium, trapezoid, capitate and hamate.

On the lateral view the distal radius should align with the lunate, and the capitate should sit in the concavity of the lunate.

Bones
Trace the contour of the bones looking for cortical breaks. A bony flake lying posterior to the carpus on the lateral view usually represents a triquetral fracture.

Cartilage and joints
The intercarpal joint spaces are usually less than 2 mm. Widening suggests ligamentous injury.

Soft tissues
Soft tissue swelling may be present at the site of injury.

Distal radius and ulna fractures
Fractures of the distal radius and/or the ulna, account for around 75% of wrist bony injuries. Most fractures occur as a result of a fall on the outstretched, pronated hand with impact on the palm. Young children tend to sustain greenstick fractures of the distal radius, whereas adolescents often injure the growth plate with dorsal displacement of the epiphysis. Young adults require significant force to sustain fractures, which are often comminuted and intra-articular. Older adults with weaker cortical bone, tend to sustain extra-articular fractures of the distal radius with displacement of the distal fragment.

Several classifications have been developed for distal radius injuries, which can be intra- or extra-articular, and simple or comminuted. Fractures with an offset of more than 1 mm in any plane, including the articular surface, are considered displaced. The severity of injury can be judged by the degree of displacement and comminution, and the presence of joint extension. Distal radial fractures with more than 5 mm of shortening tend to be unstable. Comminuted, displaced or intra-articular fractures may require CT to help plan treatment. Fractures of the distal radius can result

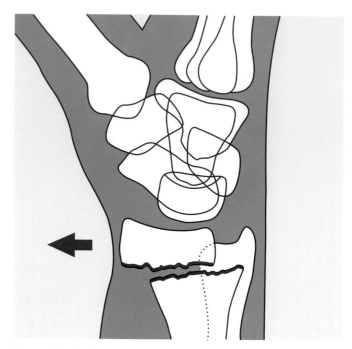

Figure 9.19 Line drawing illustrating a Smith fracture of the distal radius.

in injury to the median nerve or sensory branch of the radial nerve. Around 60% of distal radius fractures are associated with fractures of the ulnar styloid.

The term "Colles fracture" classically describes an extra-articular distal radius fracture occurring within 4 cm of the articular surface of the radius. The term is now loosely applied to any distal radius fracture with dorsal displacement of the fracture fragments.

A fall on to the supinated hand may result in the Smith fracture (Figure 9.19), which is a transverse fracture of the distal radial metaphysis with palmar displacement of the fragment. This is also referred to as a reverse Colles fracture.

The dorsal Barton fracture is an intra-articular fracture of the dorsal margin of the distal radius with dorsal displacement of the carpus (Figure 9.20a). An intra-articular fracture, with volar displacement is referred to as volar Barton fracture (Figure 9.20b).

The Hutchinson fracture, otherwise known as the "chauffeur fracture", is an intra-articular fracture involving the radial styloid process extending into the radiocarpal articulation.

Carpal fractures
The scaphoid is the most commonly injured carpal bone, with fractures involving the tubercle, distal pole, waist or proximal pole. A dedicated "scaphoid series" of radiographs should be performed including dorsopalmar, dorsopalmar with ulnar deviation, lateral and oblique projections. In the context of major wrist trauma, scaphoid fractures are often associated with other fractures or dislocations, which tend to occur in a zone of vulnerability defined by the lesser and greater arcs. The greater arc passes through the radial styloid, scaphoid, capitate and ulnar styloid. The lesser arc courses around the lunate. If there is clinical suspicion of a scaphoid fracture and initial radiographs are normal, then immobilization and

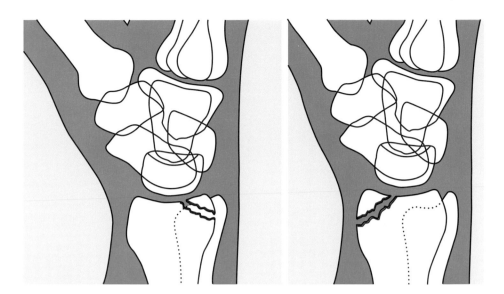

Figure 9.20 Line drawings illustrating (a) a dorsal Barton fracture and (b) a volar Barton fracture.

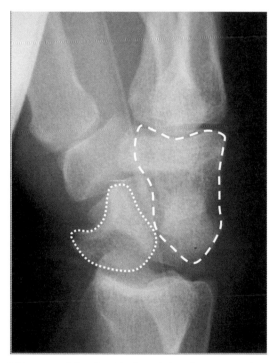

Figure 9.21 Lunate dislocation. The lateral view demonstrates the relative positions of the lunate (dotted line) and capitate (dashed line). Radiolunate alignment is disrupted. Compare with Figure 9.19.

follow-up is essential. MRI or a nuclear medicine bone scan can be helpful in these cases.

Carpal dislocations

Carpal dislocations are uncommon and are described in relation to the lunate. With lunate dislocation the lunate has a triangular appearance on the AP view, with loss of normal carpal alignment. On the lateral view the lunate demonstrates volar displacement and rotation. The position of the capitate remains unchanged (Figure 9.21).

With perilunate dislocation the lunate may be normally aligned or volarly displaced and the capitate is dorsally displaced. This injury is often associated with a scaphoid fracture, an injury known as the trans-scaphoid perilunate dislocation (Figure 9.22).

Scaphoid dislocation is a very uncommon injury that may occur in isolation or in association with disruption of the distal carpal row.

Hand injury

The hand is a common site of injury and there are a variety of fractures, avulsions and dislocations that will not be discussed in detail.

Dislocations of the carpometacarpal joints are relatively uncommon but significant injuries, often in association with metacarpal base and distal carpal row fractures. These dislocations are usually dorsal and may be difficult to recognize on DP or oblique radiographs often requiring a lateral film for confirmation. The fourth and fifth carpometacarpal joints are most frequently affected, but occasionally the second and third are also involved (Figure 9.23). CT is often helpful to assess these injuries.

Intra-articular fractures of the first metacarpal should be differentiated from extra-articular fractures, as the former will usually require surgical fixation. Bennett's fracture is an intra-articular fracture-dislocation of the base of the first metacarpal. Typically there is a small fragment at the base that remains in articulation with the trapezium with the remainder of the metacarpal dislocated dorsally. The Rolando fracture is a comminuted Bennett's fracture.

Traumatic amputation

Traumatic amputation of all or part of the upper limb can result from a variety of mechanisms. The amputated part may provide a valuable source of tissue, even if it is not fully replantable. Radiography of the residual limb and amputated portion should

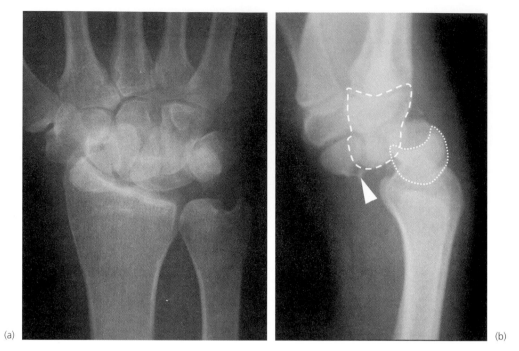

(a)　　　　　　　　　　　　　　　　　　　　　　　　(b)

Figure 9.22 Trans-scaphoid perilunate dislocation. (a) The AP view shows overlap of the proximal and distal carpal rows. (b) The lateral view demonstrates the relative positions of the lunate (dotted line) and capitate (dashed line). There is a displaced scaphoid fracture (arrowhead). Radiolunate alignment is maintained.

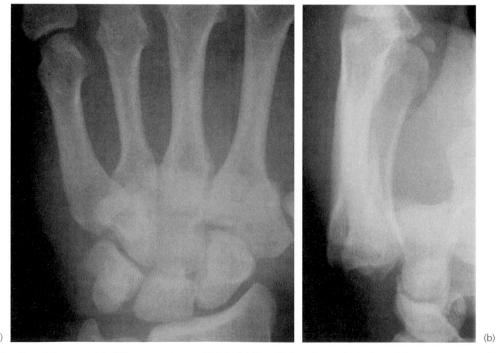

(a)　　　　　　　　　　　　　　　　　　　　　　　　(b)

Figure 9.23 Dorsal dislocation of the second to fifth carpometacarpal joints. (a) The AP view demonstrates loss of the carpometacarpal joint spaces with bony overlap. (b) The lateral view confirms dorsal dislocation.

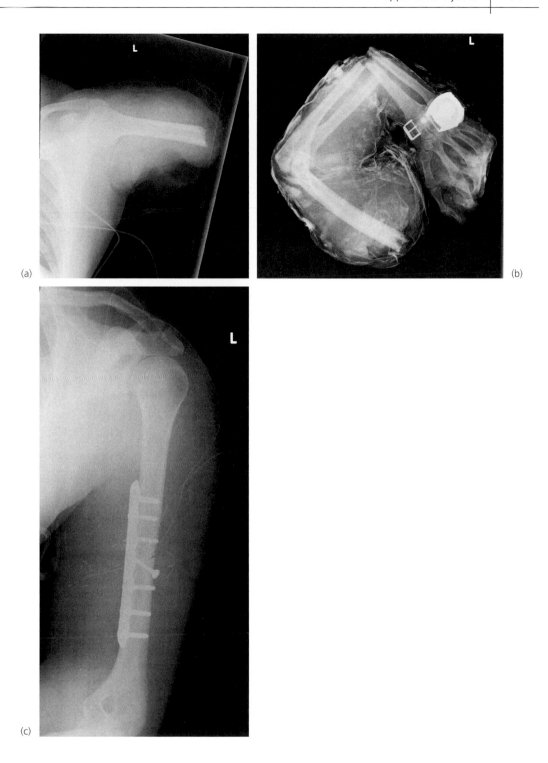

Figure 9.24 Traumatic amputation through the humerus. (a) The AP view of the residual limb demonstrates a clean fracture line with no radio-opaque loose bodies. (b) The amputated portion demonstrates a fracture of the forearm. (c) The replanted limb is demonstrated.

be performed to determine the level of injury, the bone status and the presence of foreign material (Figure 9.24).

Further reading

Bohndorf K & Kilcoyne RF. Traumatic injuries: imaging of peripheral musculoskeletal injuries. *European Radiology* 2002; **12**: 1605–1616.

Chan O. *ABC of Emergency Radiology*. Blackwell, Oxford, 2007.

Goss TP. Double disruptions of the superior shoulder suspensory complex. *Journal of Orthopaedic Trauma* 1993; **7**: 99–106.

Pretorius ES & Fishman EK. Volume-rendered three-dimensional spiral CT: musculoskeletal applications. *Radiographics* 1999; **19**: 1143–1160.

Sonin A. Fractures of the elbow and forearm. *Seminars in Musculoskeletal Radiology* 2000; **4**: 171–191.

CHAPTER 10

Lower Limb Injuries

David Elias[1] and Richard A. Schaefer[2]

[1]King's College Hospital, London, UK
[2]Uniformed Services University of the Health Sciences, Bethesda, MD, USA

OVERVIEW

- Management of lower limb injury should be incorporated into the "ABCDE" approach to trauma
- Injuries with potential neurovascular injury may require emergency management prior to radiography (e.g. ankle dislocations must be reduced urgently)
- Bony injuries require two, ideally orthogonal, radiographic views and the joints above and below a fracture must be included
- Computed tomography (CT) is often required for further evaluation in hip, knee and ankle/ foot fractures. CT angiography is mandatory where there is risk of associated vascular injury
- Magnetic resonance imaging may be valuable for assessing ligamentous injury in knee or ankle trauma but should be delayed until patients are stable

Introduction

The initial evaluation of lower limb injuries in the context of poly-trauma should be incorporated into the "ABCDE" approach to trauma management. A clinically apparent lower limb long bone fracture may account for significant blood loss and splinting at an early stage will aid haemostasis and pain relief. Radiographic imaging will be required before definitive treatment, but should not delay emergency management of clinically obvious injuries such as ankle dislocations, which require urgent reduction to prevent neurovascular injury and maintain foot viability.

An understanding of common lower limb injury patterns enables early recognition of those injuries likely to be complicated by neurovascular damage, which need urgent clinical and imaging assessment prior to definitive treatment. Additionally an appreciation of commonly associated injuries will prevent clinically occult injuries from being missed. For example, calcaneal fractures following a fall should prompt a search for an associated thoracolumbar spine fracture.

ABC of Imaging in Trauma. By Leonard J. King and David C. Wherry
Published 2010 by Blackwell Publishing

As with all skeletal trauma, lower limb injuries require at least two, ideally orthogonal, radiographic views. For hip injuries the anteroposterior (AP) view should be supplemented with either a shoot through or frog-leg lateral. Lateral knee radiographs in trauma should be performed as horizontal beam films to enable identification of a lipohaemarthrosis (fat–fluid level). AP and lateral ankle radiographs may be supplemented with a 15–20 degree internal oblique mortice view to identify malalignments. Foot radiographs should include dorsoplantar (DP), oblique and lateral views. The presence of a long bone fracture necessitates radiographs of the joints above and below the injury as there is a frequent association of further injuries at these sites.

Computed tomography (CT) is helpful in the evaluation of complex bony anatomy such as the acetabulum, tibial plateau, midfoot and hindfoot, which may be poorly seen on conventional radiographs, and can assist with surgical planning. Magnetic resonance imaging (MRI) is also valuable to assess associated ligament, tendon or cartilage injury, but is usually delayed until patients have been adequately stabilized.

Hip injuries

Hip dislocations are relatively uncommon injuries usually seen in the context of severe trauma such as motor vehicle accidents. Dislocations may be anterior, posterior, central or, rarely, inferior. Posterior dislocations account for 85–90% of cases and typically occur when a posteriorly directed force is applied to the knee with the hip in flexion, such as when the knee strikes the dashboard of a car. In most cases there is an associated fracture of the posterior acetabular rim. Femoral head fractures are less common.

Posterior dislocations are usually evident on AP radiographs with obvious superior displacement of the femoral head. Direct posterior dislocations may be more subtle on AP radiographs with only slight loss of congruence of the hip joint and non-visualization of the lesser trochanter due to internal rotation of the femur. Distinction between a posterior dislocation and the much less common anterosuperior dislocation may be difficult on the AP radiograph alone. In posterior dislocations the femur is adducted and internally rotated such that the lesser trochanter is obscured (Figure 10.1), while in anterior dislocations the femur is abducted and externally rotated prominently profiling the lesser trochanter. A lateral view is confirmatory.

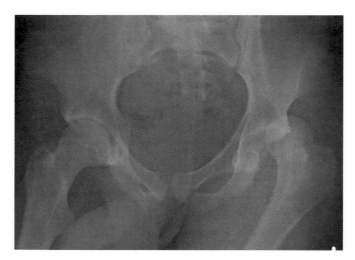

Figure 10.1 Anteroposterior pelvic radiograph demonstrating posterior dislocation of the left hip.

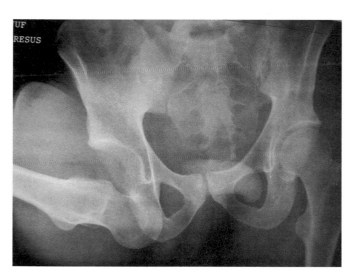

Figure 10.2 Anteroposterior pelvic radiograph demonstrating antero-inferior dislocation of the right hip.

Posterior dislocations are commonly associated with femoral fractures, usually in the mid-shaft but they may be supracondylar or subtrochanteric. After reduction of hip dislocations, persisting incongruity of the hip joint or widening by comparison with the contralateral hip may indicate failed reduction or the presence of interposed fracture fragments or soft tissue within the joint.

Anterior dislocations account for around 11% of hip dislocations following forced abduction plus external rotation of the thigh, and are classified into superior and inferior types (Figure 10.2). The femoral head may come to rest over the obturator foramen, below the anterior superior iliac spine, or rarely in the perineum. Associated femoral head fractures are common, while acetabular rim fractures are less common.

CT is essential in the management of hip dislocations. The presence of femoral or acetabular fractures causing joint incongruity or instability, central acetabular fractures or intra-articular bone fragments can all be identified with CT and will mandate open rather than closed reduction.

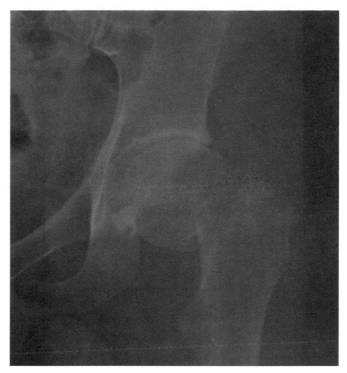

Figure 10.3 Anteroposterior radiograph of the left hip in a young adult male demonstrating a traumatic intra-articular fracture of the left femoral neck.

Complications of hip dislocation include:
- sciatic nerve palsy 10–13% of posterior dislocations – usually transient
- peri-articular calcification
- avascular necrosis of the femoral head
- recurrent dislocation – especially with a significant posterior acetabular rim fragment
- hip osteoarthritis.

Femoral fractures

Most femoral neck fractures occur in elderly patients following minor trauma and are generally associated with osteoporosis. Major trauma in young patients with normal bone density is more likely to cause hip dislocation or a femoral shaft fracture, but femoral neck fractures can occasionally occur (Figure 10.3). Femoral neck fractures are divided into intra- and extracapsular types (Figure 10.4). Intracapsular neck fractures can be classified according to the Garden system (Figure 10.5). Intracapsular fractures may be associated with disruption of synovial epiphyseal vessels, which form the predominant blood supply to the femoral head. Thus the risk of avascular necrosis is up to 30% in displaced subcapital fractures. Non-union occurs in up to 25% of displaced intracapsular fractures. Other complications include DVT, malunion, osteoarthritis or femoral neck osteolysis.

Intertrochanteric fractures are extracapsular and frequently comminuted. Fractures with an increasing number of fragments are more likely to be unstable. Subtrochanteric fractures (including intertrochanteric fractures that extend to the subtrochanteric region) may occur as a result of severe trauma and are inherently unstable (Figure 10.6).

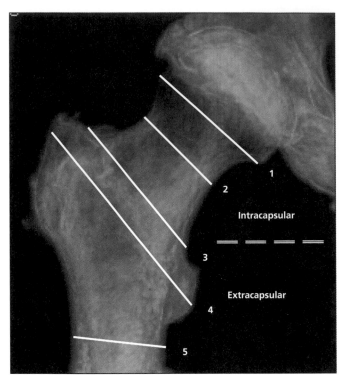

Figure 10.4 Diagram demonstrating the anatomical subtypes of proximal femoral fractures.
1. Subcapital
2. Transcervical
3. Basicervical
4. Intertrochanteric
5. Subtrochanteric

Subcapital, transcervical and basicervical fractures are intracapsular. The others are extracapsular.

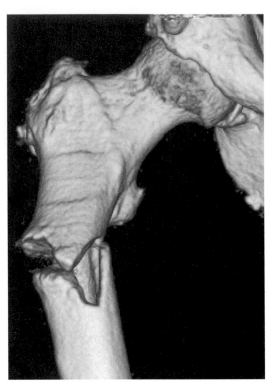

Figure 10.6 Three-dimensional volume-rendered CT reconstruction of a comminuted subtrochanteric fracture of the left femur.

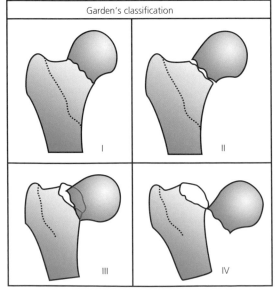

Type Description
- 1 Incomplete, undisplaced, including valgus impacted
- 2 Complete, undisplaced
- 3 Complete, partial displacement
- 4 Complete, total displacement with loss of contact between fracture fragments

Figure 10.5 Diagram illustrating the Garden classification of intracapsular femoral neck fractures.

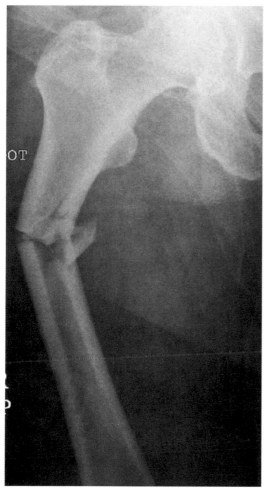

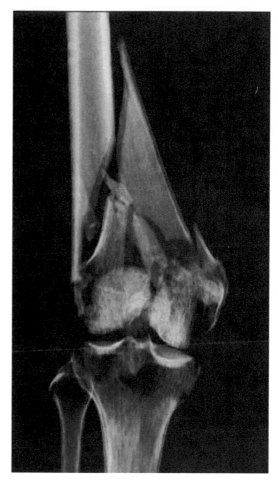

Figure 10.7 Anteroposterior radiograph of a proximal femoral shaft fracture with abduction of the proximal fragment.

Figure 10.8 Three-dimensional volume-rendered CT reconstruction of a comminuted supracondylar fracture of the right femur.

Femoral shaft fractures usually require severe forces and typically occur in motor vehicle collisions. Around 20% are associated with other ipsilateral injuries, typically of the hip or knee, and radiographs of the pelvis and knee are mandatory. The proximal femoral fragment is usually abducted (Figure 10.7) and adduction of the proximal fragment should raise the possibility of an associated hip dislocation. Ligamentous knee injuries occur in 17–33% of patients with femoral shaft fracture and may be occult due to difficulties with clinical examination of the knee in these patients. MRI is helpful in these circumstances.

Supracondylar fractures have a variety of different configurations. Evidence of intra-articular extension should be sought as this necessitates open reduction and internal fixation (Figure 10.8). The distal fragment may be angulated by the pull of gastrocnemius and displacement can result in popliteal artery injury in 2–3% of cases.

Knee injuries

Knee trauma can produce an extensive range of bony and soft tissue injuries. Shearing or rotatory forces directed at the articular surface of a femoral condyle may produce an osteochondral frac-

ture. These are often occult on conventional radiographs but there may be irregularity of the articular surface and intra-articular bone fragments.

Tibial plateau fractures (Figure 10.9) occur most commonly in females over 50 years of age, usually following twisting falls. Typically there is a valgus force with impaction of the femoral condyle on the plateau. Injury is confined to the lateral plateau in 75–80% of cases. Fewer than 25% are due to motor vehicle–pedestrian accidents, typically due to a car bumper striking the knee. These fractures are often subtle, requiring careful attention to AP and lateral radiographs for identification. A horizontal beam lateral radiograph may demonstrate a fat–fluid level within a distended suprapatellar bursa due to haemorrhage and marrow fat leaking into the joint (Figure 10.10). CT is valuable, since the degree of fracture depression determines the need for surgery and this is difficult to assess on conventional radiographs (Figure 10.11). Alternatively, MRI may be used to assess these injuries, with the advantage of demonstrating associated ligamentous and meniscal injuries, which are reported in 68–97% of cases.

Fibular head fractures may be isolated injuries due to a direct blow, but are most commonly associated with tibial plateau

Schatzker Classification for Tibial Plateau Fractures

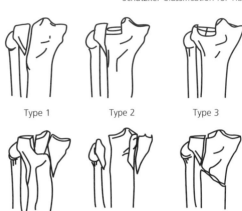

Type 1   Type 2   Type 3

Type 4   Type 5   Type 6

Type   Description
- I   Split fracture of the lateral tibial plateau
       without depression
- II   Split fracture of the lateral tibial plateau
       with depression
- III Depressed fracture
       of the lateral tibial plateau without split
- IV   Medial tibial plateau fracture of
       any type (may also involve the tibial spines)
- V   Split medial and lateral tibial
       plateau fractures (bicondylar). Metaphysis is
       still in continuity with the diaphysis
- VI   Metaphyseal fracture that
       separates the articular surface from the diaphysis

Figure 10.9 Diagram illustrating the Schatzker classification of tibial plateau fractures.

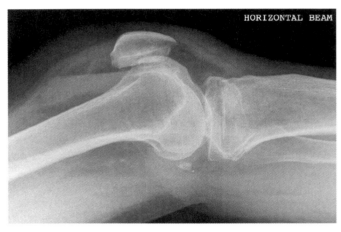

HORIZONTAL BEAM

Figure 10.10 Horizontal beam lateral knee radiograph demonstrating a large joint effusion with a fat–fluid level and a tibial plateau fracture.

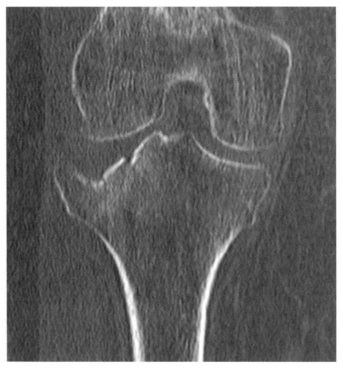

Figure 10.11 Coronal reformat CT scan image of a depressed lateral tibial plateau fracture.

fractures. Fractures of the fibular neck or proximal shaft may be part of a Maisonneuve pattern with an associated ankle injury.

Patella fractures may be due to a direct blow or to excessive quadriceps contraction with the knee fixed in flexion (Figure 10.12). Fractures may be transverse, vertical or comminuted, with or without displacement. Patellar dislocation is almost always in the lateral direction and classically occurs in teenage girls. Usually dislocation is transient and the presentation is with a non-specific acute haemarthrosis. In many patients dislocation becomes recurrent. Radiographs following injury rarely show a dislocated patella (Figure 10.13). More commonly a skyline view shows osteochondral injury with separated fragments from the medial aspect of the patella and/or the anterior tip of the lateral femoral condyle, due to impaction during dislocation. These fractures can be confirmed with CT or MRI (Figure 10.14).

Dislocation of the knee is uncommon and may be anterior, posterior, medial, lateral or rotational. The risk of associated popliteal artery and peroneal nerve injury is significant (Figure 10.15). Urgent CT angiography should be performed following reduction of the dislocation, as associated popliteal artery injury needs prompt recognition and treatment. Typically, there is also rupture of at least three major knee ligaments and MRI is valuable to assess

this after the dislocation has been reduced and any vascular injury addressed (Figure 10.16). MRI can be complicated by the presence of a conventional external fixator, the metallic components of which will demonstrate strong magnetic attraction and generate induction currents, causing heating with the risk of thermal injury. However, MR-compatible external fixators which can be safely imaged are now commercially available.

Injury to the knee ligaments usually results in clinical signs of instability and a knee effusion. Avulsion fractures occasionally provide relatively specific evidence of particular ligamentous injuries on conventional radiographs. For example, the Segond fracture, which is a small avulsion fragment of the lateral margin of the tibial plateau is associated with anterior cruciate ligament (ACL)

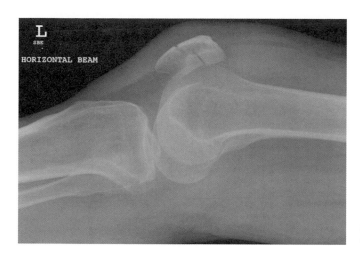

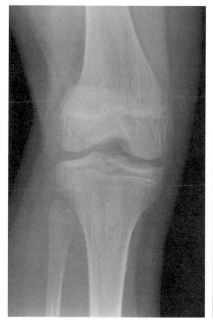

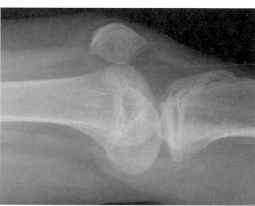

Figure 10.12 Horizontal beam lateral radiograph showing a transverse fracture of the patella and a fat-fluid level.

Figure 10.13 AP and lateral radiographs of a right knee demonstrating lateral dislocation of the patella.

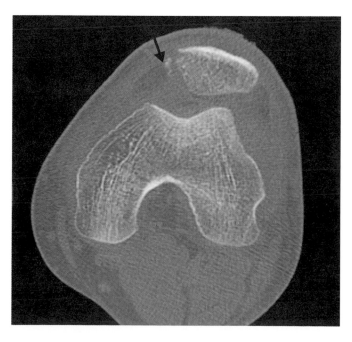

Figure 10.14 Axial CT image of the left knee following lateral dislocation demonstrating an avulsion fracture of the medial patella (arrow) and persistent lateral patella subluxation.

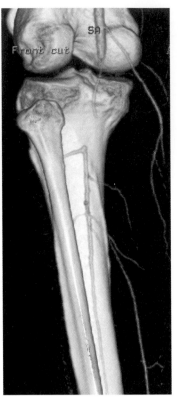
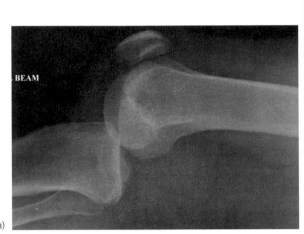

(a)

(b)

Figure 10.15 (a) Lateral radiograph demonstrating posterior knee dislocation. (b) Subsequent CT angiogram following reduction demonstrates occlusion of the popliteal artery.

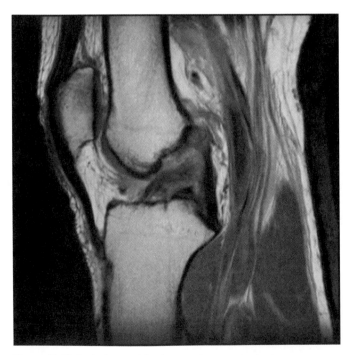

Figure 10.16 Sagittal T1 weighted magnetic resonance image demonstrating rupture of the anterior and posterior cruciate ligaments following knee dislocation.

injury in over 75% of cases. ACL injury may also cause avulsion of the anterior tibial eminence, usually in children. Avulsion of the fibular styloid process may be seen in fibular collateral ligament injury. Avulsion fractures of the superior or inferior patellar pole or the tibial tuberosity may be seen in extensor mechanism injuries.

Tibial fractures

Tibial shaft fractures usually affect the middle or distal third of the bone and there is usually an associated fibular fracture (Figure 10.17). There is a significant association with ipsilateral fracture dislocation of the hip or fracture of the femur, and pelvic plus femoral radiographs should therefore be obtained. Complications of tibial fractures include compartment syndrome, delayed union, non-union and re-fracture.

Ankle injuries

While most ankle fractures are readily identified on conventional radiographs, the presence of ligamentous injury may need to be inferred by malalignments on static radiographs or stress views. The lateral clear space is the distance between the medial border of the lateral malleolus and the base of the fibular notch of the lateral tibia. Where this is wider than 5 mm (or 2 mm wider than the asymptomatic ankle), syndesmotic rupture is inferred. Widening of the medial clear space of more than 3–4 mm between the medial border of the talus and the medial malleolus suggests deltoid ligament rupture

Certain injury patterns are particularly associated with major trauma. Axial ankle compression injuries after a fall from height or a high-speed motor vehicle collision may produce pronation–dorsiflexion or pilon fractures. In this injury the talus is driven proximally and, with increasing force, there is a progression of injuries from medial malleolar fracture (stage 1), to avulsion of the anterior lip of the tibial plafond (stage 2) to fracture of the supramalleolar fibula (stage 3) and finally transverse fracture of the dorsal tibia above the plafond (stage 4). The tibial plafond may be markedly comminuted with peripheral displacement of fragments and proximal talar migration. CT demonstrates the bony fragments most clearly and is indicated preoperatively (Figure 10.18). Pilon fractures should be distinguished from the more common trimalleolar fractures. The latter show no fracture of the anterior lip of the tibial plafond, which is a hallmark of the pilon fracture. Trimalleolar fractures occur with external rotation of the foot and typically represent unstable fracture dislocations. Pure ankle dislocations without fracture are uncommon but may be seen in young adults, particularly with open injury. The talus usually displaces medially and neurovascular injury is common.

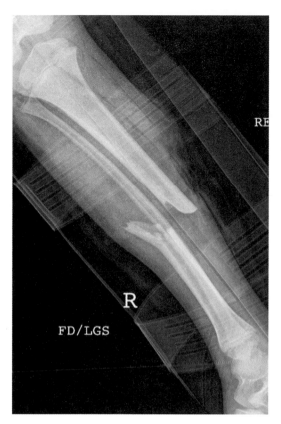

Figure 10.17 Radiograph of the right lower leg demonstrating mid-shaft fractures of the tibia and fibula with external rotation.

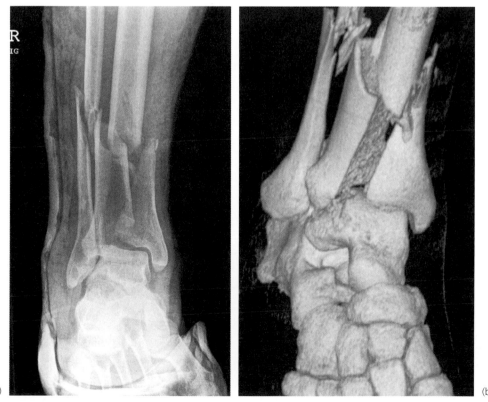

(a) (b)

Figure 10.18 (a) Plain radiograph and (b) three-dimensional volume-rendered CT reconstruction demonstrating a comminuted pilon fracture of the distal tibia.

Foot injuries

Talus

Fractures of the talus can involve the head, neck or body, including osteochondral injuries of the talar dome and fractures of the lateral or posterior process. Talar neck fractures classically occur after head-on motor vehicle collisions when the foot is jammed against the brake pedal (Figure 10.19). These are usually vertical fractures in the coronal plane and around half are associated with either tibiotalar or subtalar dislocation (Box 10.1). Talar neck fractures, and especially fracture dislocations, may be complicated by avascular necrosis of the talar body.

Subtalar joint

Subtalar dislocation can occur when falling from a height on to the inverted foot. This may present as a pure subtalar dislocation with only mild talonavicular or calcaneocuboid subluxation, or as a medial swivel dislocation, in which the navicular is medially dislo-

cated and there is relatively mild subtalar and calcaneocuboid subluxation. CT is helpful especially in identifying commonly associated talar fractures. Mid-tarsal or Chopart dislocations in which there is talonavicular and calcaneocuboid dislocation with a congruent subtalar joint are less common (Figure 10.20).

Calcaneum

Compression fractures of the calcaneum are usually sustained as a result of falling from a height. They may be bilateral and are associated with spinal compression fractures, particularly at the thoracolumbar junction. Compressive calcaneal fractures generally involve the subtalar joint with some depression of the posterior facet. Böhler's angle is reduced from its normal value of 20–40 degrees (Figure 10.21). These fractures are often highly comminuted and CT is helpful in identifying the multiple fragments and their posi-

---

Box 10.1 **Modified Hawkins classification of talar neck fractures**

Type	Description
I	Undisplaced fracture
II	Displaced fracture + subluxation/dislocation of subtalar joint
III	Displaced fracture + dislocation of subtalar and tibiotalar joints
IV	Displaced fracture as in III + disruption of talonavicular joint

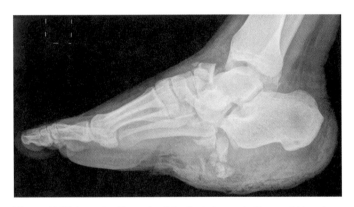

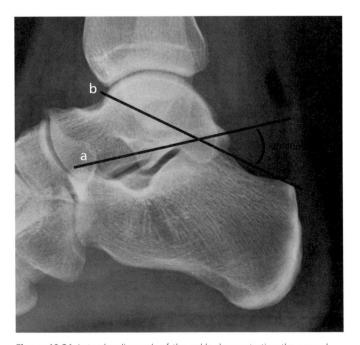

Figure 10.20 Lateral radiograph of the foot demonstrating a mid-tarsal (chopart) fracture dislocation.

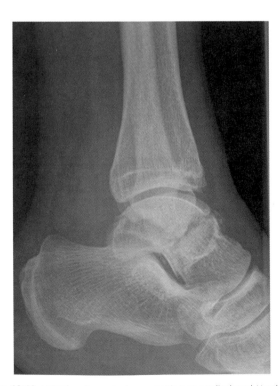

Figure 10.19 Lateral radiograph demonstrating an undisplaced Hawkins type 1 fracture of the talar neck.

Figure 10.21 Lateral radiograph of the ankle demonstrating the normal Böhlers's angle.

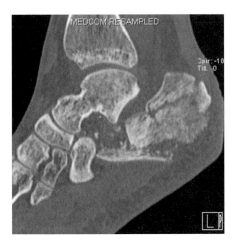

Figure 10.22 Sagittal CT reconstruction demonstrating a comminuted intra-articular fracture of the calcaneum.

Box 10.2 **Sanders classification for intra-articular calcaneal fractures**

Type	Description
1	No significant displacement (<2 mm)
2	Single displaced intra-articular fracture on coronal CT of the posterior facet resulting in two large fragments
3	Two displaced intra-articular fractures on coronal CT of the posterior facet resulting in two large fragments
4	More than two displaced fracture lines resulting in further comminution

---

tions (Figure 10.22) allowing fracture classification (Box 10.2). There may be associated subluxation/dislocation of the peroneal tendons or impingement/entrapment of the peroneal or flexor hallucis longus tendons by bone spikes. These changes are shown to advantage on CT or MRI.

Tarsometatarsal joints

Fracture dislocations of the tarsometatarsal joints (Lisfranc dislocation) are encountered in motor vehicle accidents or in injuries where the weight of the body rotates about a fixed forefoot. Lisfranc dislocations are classified as homolateral if the metatarsals (usually all five) sublux laterally, and divergent if the first metatarsal subluxes medially and the remainder laterally (Figure 10.23). These injuries may be subtle or even occult on conventional radiographs. In the presence of mid-foot soft tissue swelling, the DP radiograph should be carefully examined for subtle malalignment between the lateral border of the first metatarsal and the lateral border of the medial cuneiform, and between the medial border of the second metatarsal and the medial border of the intermediate cuneiform. Similar alignments should be examined at the third and fourth tarsometatarsal joint on the oblique view. The most constant abnormality is injury at the second tarsometatarsal joint and there is usually a fracture of the second metatarsal

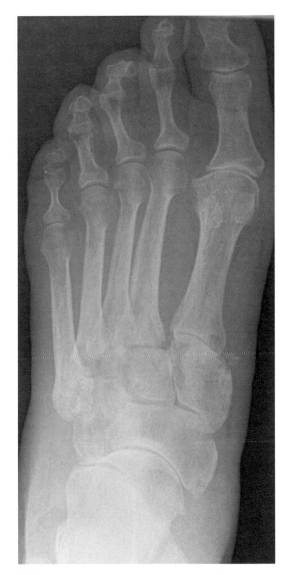

Figure 10.23 Plain radiograph of the foot demonstrating a Lis Franc injury with lateral subluxation of the second to fifth toes and multiple associated fractures.

base. There are also usually multiple small tarsometatarsal avulsion fractures and often a fracture of the cuboid. CT is usually required to identify the extent of injury and is mandatory where the diagnosis is in the doubt, as these injuries are unstable and usually require internal fixation. MRI can also be useful for demonstrating subtle injuries and can demonstrate tears of the Lis Franc ligament.

Traumatic amputation

Traumatic lower limb amputation is occasionally seen following blast injuries, motor vehicle accidents or industrial injuries. Amputation may be partial or complete and occurs at tibial level more commonly than femoral level. Immediate concerns include control of bleeding and prevention of shock. Radiography is required to assess bony injury (Figure 10.24).

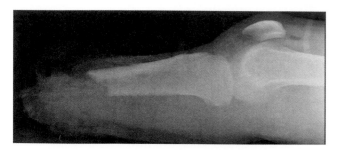

Figure 10.24 Lateral radiograph of the lower leg demonstrating a traumatic amputation.

Further reading

Rogers LF. *Radiology of Skeletal Trauma*. Churchill Livingstone, Edinburgh, 2002: chapters 20–23.

Matherne TH, Tivorsak T & Monu JUV. Calcaneal fractures: what the surgeon needs to know. *Current Problems in Diagnostic Radiology* 2007; **36**: 1–10.

Maripuri S, Rao P, Manoj-Thomas A & Mohanty K. The classification systems for tibial plateau fractures: how reliable are they? *Injury* 2008; **39**: 1216–1221.

Hunt SA, Ropiak C & Tejwani NC. Lisfranc joint injuries: diagnosis and treatment. *American Journal of Orthopedics* 2006; **35**: 376–385.

CHAPTER 11

Paediatric Trauma

Mark Griffiths[1] and Catherine Cord-Uday[2]

[1]Southampton University Hospitals NHS Trust, Southampton, Hampshire, UK
[2]Flinders Medical Centre, Adelaide, SA, Australia

OVERVIEW

- There are important differences in the patterns of injury seen in children compared with adults
- Imaging modalities using ionizing radiation, particularly computed tomography (CT) should be used judiciously in children
- Ultrasound can be useful in the assessment of paediatric trauma but cannot exclude significant injury with the same degree of accuracy as CT
- Peripheral limb injuries can result in damage to unfused growth plates and apophyses

---

Imaging of the injured child requires recognition of injury patterns that are different to those occurring in adult patients. Body proportions are different in children and the immature skeleton reacts differently to traumatic forces, with buckle and greenstick fractures. Significant visceral injury can occur in the absence of bony injury, and if a significant skeletal injury has occurred then the index of suspicion for internal injury should be high.

The injured child presents difficulties in clinical assessment and challenges in the production of diagnostic images. The ALARA (as low as reasonably achievable) principle of radiation exposure should always be adhered to in the imaging of children, who are more susceptible than adults, with an increased cancer risk for the same radiation burden. The lifetime risk of fatal malignancy following exposure to an effective radiation dose of 1 Sv is estimated at 10% in childhood compared to 5% in 20- to 60-year-olds. Decisions regarding imaging studies should where possible take account of the mechanism of injury and the clinical assessment of the injured child. The mechanism of injury should also be correlated with the injuries that are observed to ensure that the pattern is appropriate and a non-accidental injury is not overlooked. Patient movement will degrade computed tomography (CT) or magnetic resonance (MR) images and cause artefacts, which can

be a problem with young children and older children who are uncooperative due to altered mental status (Figure 11.1).

Head injury

Assessment of neurological status may be difficult in the injured child. Many of the considerations relating to cranial trauma imaging for adults may be applied to the paediatric age group; however, head injury in younger children is affected by the relatively large mass of the head compared to the rest of the body, with associated poorly developed supporting musculature. The brain thus may be exposed to increased shearing forces compared to an adult with the same mechanism of injury.

The development of the skull enables depression without fracture, and the presence of sutures enables intracranial mass effect to be tempered by sutural separation. The mid-face development also leads to greater numbers of upper compared to lower facial fractures in children. CT scanning is the mainstay of acute intracranial imaging (Figure 11.2), with plain skull films being reserved for the assessment of non-accidental injury.

Thoracic injury

Plain chest radiographs are still the mainstay of thoracic trauma imaging (Figure 11.3a). Ultrasound can be used to assess for the presence of a pericardial or pleural effusion and to demonstrate pneumothoraces, which may be occult on plain chest radiographs. Acute rib fractures may be extremely difficult to visualize on plain films, and ultrasound can also be used to show a subperiosteal haematoma or cortical step. CT can also be useful to demonstrate subtle pneumothoraces or to assist in the positioning of chest drains, and with contrast enhancement may be used to delineate vascular anatomy. Aortic injury is extremely rare in children, but in the presence of an abnormal mediastinal contour following chest trauma, it should be excluded by CT. Pulmonary haemorrhage or parenchymal contusion not visible on chest x-ray may also be demonstrated on cross-sectional imaging (Figure 11.3b).

Abdominal injury

Investigation of abdominal trauma is dependent on patient status. The haemodynamically unstable patient with obvious abdominal

ABC of Imaging in Trauma. By Leonard J. King and David C. Wherry
Published 2010 by Blackwell Publishing

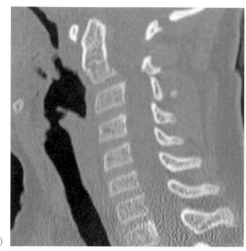
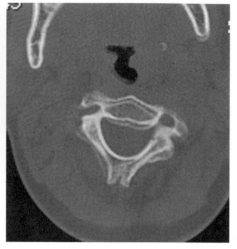

(a)
(b)

Figure 11.1 CT scan images of the cervical spine in a child following trauma. An apparent C2 fracture on the sagittal reformat image (a) is due to motion artefact, which can be clearly recognised on the axial plane image (b).

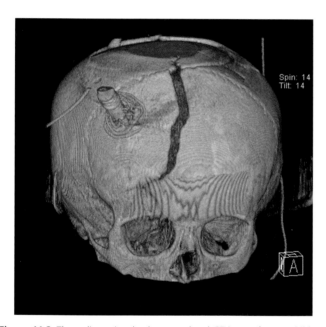

Figure 11.2 Three-dimensional volume-rendered CT image from a child with a severe head injury demonstrating a depressed fracture of the vertex and a vertical fracture of the frontal bone. An intracranial pressure bolt is in situ.

injury or intraperitoneal free fluid identified on abdominal ultrasound should undergo laparotomy.

Ultrasound should be the initial investigation of choice when examining children. There is no radiation burden to the patient and the investigation can be repeated if the clinical status changes. Ultrasound is sensitive to the presence of free intraperitoneal fluid but is less specific than CT for solid organ injury in most reported studies. Many studies, however, rely on a focused assessment of sonography in trauma (FAST) examination of the abdomen for assessment, and a more thorough abdominal examination by an experienced operator can increase the sensitivity and specificity for

visceral injury. Ultrasound examination can be performed at the bedside without the need for patient preparation or administration of intravenous contrast and concurrently with other procedures. Colour-flow imaging can be used to assess organ perfusion and may demonstrate pseudoaneurysm formation. Localized collections are an indicator of adjacent injury, for example a sentinel clot related to a splenic injury or focal haematoma adjacent to a fracture. Ultrasound cannot, however, reliably demonstrate visceral injuries such as lacerations, pelvicaliceal injury or localized bowel perforation. Ultrasound examination should therefore be used in conjunction with clinical evaluation and observation, with the use of repeat scans to reassess if the signs or symptoms change. Clinical assessment cannot be replaced by a single ultrasound examination.

CT examination of the abdomen with a modern multidetector scanner is a relatively quick procedure. Intravenous contrast enhancement is required for assessment of solid organ injury and vascular anatomy. Scans are normally performed in the portal venous phase of enhancement for optimal assessment of parenchymal injury; however, arterial phase scanning is useful in the assessment of arterial injury, which may be amenable to minimally invasive therapy. CT examination of the abdomen should include the pelvis to exclude free fluid as this is the most dependent portion of the peritoneal cavity in the supine position. Oral contrast may be used but bowel opacification is often limited in children and modern thin-slice imaging technology provides three-dimensional evaluation to aid assessment of bowel injury without the necessity for oral contrast. Extraluminal oral contrast is a reliable indicator of bowel injury, but its absence has poor negative predictive value. CT scanning will demonstrate free intraperitoneal gas as a sign of bowel perforation, but bowel injury may occur without free gas and air may track into the abdomen from a pneumomediastinum or pneumothorax mimicking a bowel injury.

Although CT can produce a rapid and accurate radiological diagnosis, the clinical impact of this to the patient has to be coun-

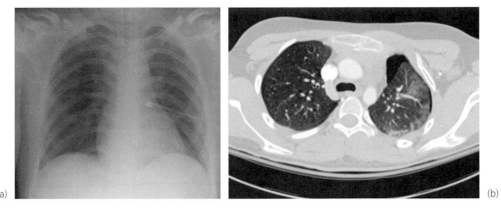

Figure 11.3 (a) Chest radiograph and (b) CT scan of a child with blunt trauma to the chest. There are bilateral clavicle fractures, rib fractures and a left apical pneumothorax. The CT also demonstrates pulmonary contusion and a sternal fracture.

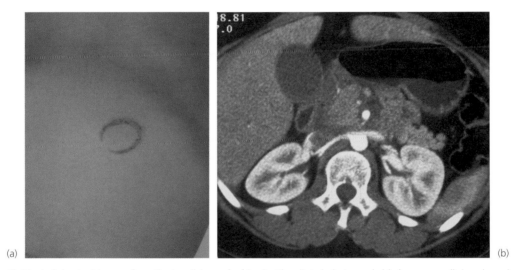

Figure 11.4 Child with blunt abdominal trauma from the handlebars of a bicycle. The clinical photograph (a) shows a small ring shaped contusion. Subsequent abdominal CT (b) demonstrates pancreatic rupture.

tered by the radiation dose being delivered. Studies have shown an increasing use of CT, with relatively low yields of significant positive findings. This suggests that CT is being overused or patient selection criteria are poor. It is also important to recognize that a positive examination may not alter management in a haemodynamically stable patient, though clinician confidence is improved. Approximately 5% of patients with abnormal findings on abdominal CT proceed to surgery for these injuries, thus CT rarely changes the clinical decision for operative intervention. Laparoscopy or CT scanning is indicated in the presence of penetrating abdominal trauma.

Both the liver and spleen are frequently injured in blunt abdominal trauma, with hepatic injury having a higher mortality. The CT findings can be used to classify liver injuries into low or high grade and document portal or biliary tract injury. However, the pattern of hepatic or splenic injuries and the volume of free fluid within the peritoneum do not necessarily correlate with the need for operative intervention. Active arterial bleeding can sometimes be identified by the presence of extravasated contrast, which has a similar density to that of the aorta, and embolization or operative intervention may be of value in these cases. Compared with adults, splenic injury in children is less likely to require operative intervention.

Pancreatic injury occurs rarely, most commonly due to a handlebar (Figure 11.4) or lap belt injury. Bruising over the epigastrium is a suggestive clinical sign. Direct impact compresses the pancreas against the lumbar spine and there is often an associated duodenal injury. Early CT may miss pancreatic injury and high-resolution ultrasound examination may be of value in the presence of a raised amylase. Pancreatic injury in the absence of an appropriate history of trauma is highly suggestive of non-accidental injury. Follow-up imaging in the presence of raised amylase is warranted to exclude pseudocyst formation.

Renal injury is more common in children than adults due to their body habitus providing less protection and the relatively large size of the kidneys compared to those of adults. Patients with renal injury will most commonly have haematuria. Perfusion of the kidney can be assessed by ultrasound with colour-flow imaging. CT can be used to grade injuries from minor contusions through to shattering of the renal parenchyma; however, most renal injuries can be successfully managed non-operatively and CT grading does not correlate with requirement for intervention.

In young children the full bladder is essentially an intra-abdominal organ, making it more prone to traumatic rupture, which can produce free intra-abdominal fluid. This injury is often due to a kick or punch to the lower abdomen and may be associated with relatively little extrinsic bruising if the blow was not anticipated and the abdominal muscles did not contract.

Skeletal injury

CT of the torso for visceral injury also enables assessment of bony structures, such as the thoracolumbar spine and the pelvis. If a good-quality multidetector CT examination which covers the spine and pelvis has been undertaken, and appropriate bony algorithms plus multiplanar reformats are obtained, then additional plain films are usually not required to exclude injury.

Cervical spine

Children under the age of 9 years tend to sustain upper cervical spine injuries with increased risk of dislocations (Figure 11.5) and cord injury compared to older children, who more commonly have an adult-type lower cervical spine injury distribution (Figure 11.6). National Institute for Health and Clinical Excellence (NICE) guidelines recommend that the imaging assessment of cervical spine injury be performed according to adult protocols in patients over the age of 10. Below the age of 10, anteroposterior (AP) and lateral radiographs should initially be obtained. Areas of concern can then be further evaluated with CT, which is also recommended if there is an associated severe head injury with a Glasgow Coma Scale (GCS) score of less than 9, a strong clinical suspicion of injury despite normal radiographs or if the plain radiographs are technically inadequate. Spinal cord injury can occur without plain film abnormality (SCIWORA), and in the presence of abnormal neurology MR examination should be undertaken. Synchondroses may also require CT scanning and MR examination to exclude injury. CT should be performed using dose reduction where possible, as standard scanning parameters result in an increased effective dose by a factor of 2.3 for 0- to 1-year-olds, 1.5 for 1- to 5-year-olds and 1.2 in 5- to 10-year-olds.

Alignment of the cervical spine may show pseudosubluxation at C2–3, which is a normal variant in children (Figure 11.7) and this may be present to a lesser degree at C3–4. The posterior alignment must be checked to ensure that this is truly pseudosubluxation and not traumatic.

The presence of one vertebral injury should highlight the possibility of further injury in the remainder of the spinal column, for which imaging should be undertaken.

Peripheral skeletal injuries

The mainstay of peripheral limb fracture imaging is plain radiography; however, CT scanning can be used to define fragment orientation and the relationship to growth plates or articular surfaces (Figure 11.8). Scanning during the arterial phase of contrast enhancement can be used to assess peripheral vascular anatomy;

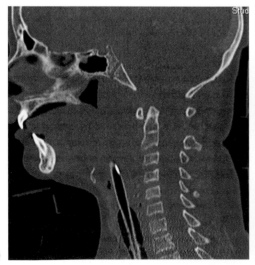
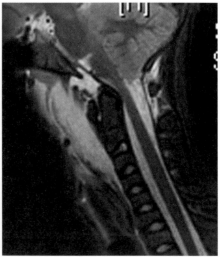

(a)　　　　　　　　　　　　　　　　(b)

Figure 11.5 Young child with traumatic atlanto-occipital dissociation. (a) Sagittal CT reconstruction demonstrates anterior subluxation of the skull base in relation to the cervical spine. (b) A sagittal short-tau inversion recovery (STIR) image from a subsequent MRI scan confirms the subluxation with ligamentous disruption and a large prevertebral haematoma.

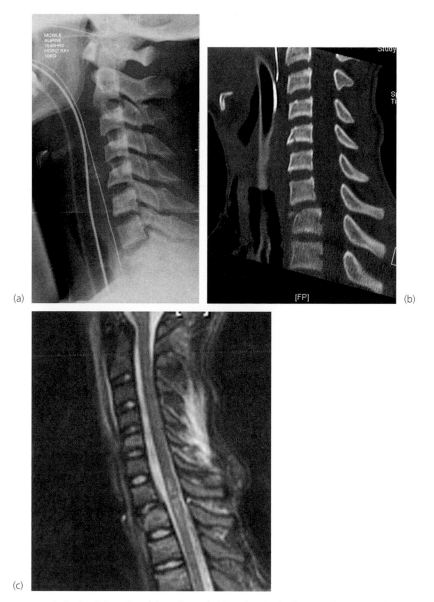

(a)

(b)

(c)

Figure 11.6 Teenager with an acute cervical spine injury. The plain radiograph (a) and sagittal reformatted CT image (b) demonstrate a compression fracture of C5 and a teardrop fracture of T1. Sagittal short-tau inversion recovery (STIR) image from a subsequent MRI scan (c) demonstrates several additional vertebral fractures, a small prevertebral haematoma, posterior interspinous ligament injury and an associated cord contusion.

however, imaging in the presence of vascular compromise should not delay operative intervention. Collateral flow in the paediatric population is extremely poor and main arterial blockage may rapidly lead to ischaemic damage (Figure 11.9). Delay due to imaging and the processing of imaging studies should not be allowed to compromise tissue viability.

In the immature skeleton ligaments are often stronger than the bones to which they are attached, and thus avulsion fractures are more common in the paediatric population. They are especially common around the pelvis in athletic adolescents (Figure 11.10). The physis represents a relatively weak region of the growing bone, and fractures involving the physes are common. They are graded according to involvement of the epiphysis and metaphysis by the Salter Harris classification (Figure 11.11), with grade I injuries having a better prognosis than the higher grades for growth plate injury (Figure 11.12) and premature fusion.

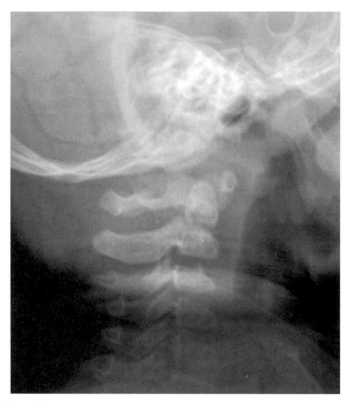

Figure 11.7 Pseudosubluxation of the C2 vertebra.

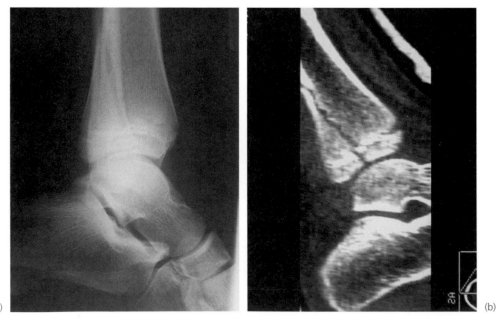

(a)

(b)

Figure 11.8 Triplane fracture of the distal tibia demonstrated on (a) a plain lateral radiograph and (b) subsequent CT, which more clearly defines the fracture pattern.

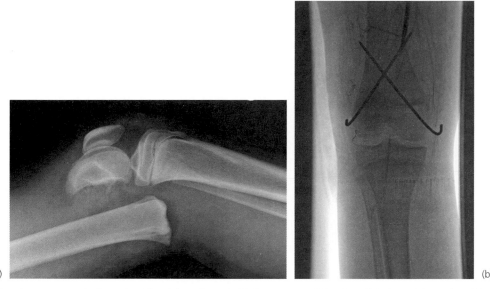

(a)　　　　　　　　　　　　　　　　　　　　(b)

Figure 11.9 Child with major trauma to the lower leg. The plain radiograph (a) demonstrates dislocation of the knee joint and avulsion of the tibial plateau epiphysis. There was an associated popliteal artery injury demonstrated on angiography that went unrecognized until after surgical intervention for the skeletal injury.

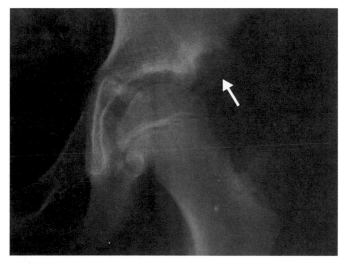

Figure 11.10 Plain radiograph of the left hip demonstrating an avulsion fracture of the anterior inferior iliac spine (arrow).

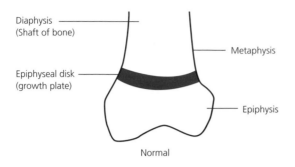

Diaphysis
(Shaft of bone)

Metaphysis

Epiphyseal disk
(growth plate)

Epiphysis

Normal

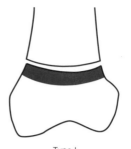

Type I

A complete physeal fracture
with or without displacement

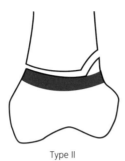

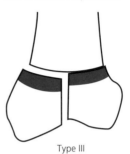

Type II

A physeal fracture that
extends through the
metaphysis, producing a chip
fracture of the metaphysis,
which may be very small

Type III

A physeal fracture that
extends through the
epiphysis

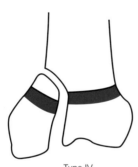

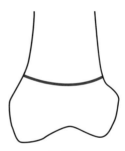

Type IV

A physeal fracture plus
epiphyseal and metaphyseal
fractures

Type V

A compression fracture of
the growth plate

Figure 11.11 The Salter Harris classification of growth plate injuries.

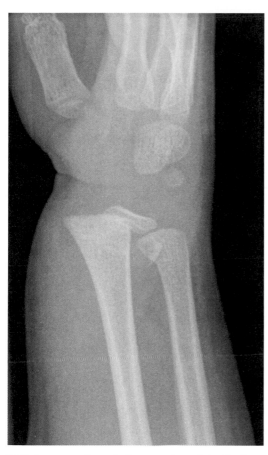

Figure 11.12 Forearm radiograph demonstrating a Salter Harris type II injury of the distal radius.

Further reading

Cartey H. *Emergency Pediatric Radiology.* Springer-Verlag, Berlin and Heidelberg, 2001.

Fenton SJ, Hansen KW, Meyers RL et al. CT scan and the pediatric trauma patient – are we overdoing it? *Journal of Pediatric Surgery* 2004; **39**: 1877–1881.

Lustrin ES *et al.* Pediatric cervical spine: normal anatomy, variants, and trauma. *Radiographics* 2003; **23**: 539–560.

National Institute for Health and Clinical Excellence. *Head Injury. Triage, assessment, investigation and early management of head injury in infants, children and adult.* NICE Clinical Guideline 56. NICE, London, 2007.

Pärtan G, Pamberger P, Blab E & Hruby W. Common tasks and problems in paediatric trauma radiology. *European Journal of Radiology* 2003; **48**: 103–124.

CHAPTER 12

Imaging Trauma in Pregnancy

Mark P. Bernstein[1] and Anne G. Rizzo[2]

[1]NYU Medical Center/Bellevue Hospital, New York, NY, USA
[2]Virginia Commonwealth University School of Medicine, Richmond, VA, USA *and* Uniformed Services University of the Health Sciences, Bethesda, MD, USA

OVERVIEW

- Trauma is the primary cause of non-obstetrical maternal mortality
- The best chance for fetal survival is maternal survival. There is seldom fetal survival without maternal survival
- Trauma in pregnancy, major or minor, is associated with increased risk of fetal demise
- Ultrasound and CT offer complementary roles in assessing fetal and maternal injuries respectively
- Diagnostic radiation doses and risks are low, and the benefits of accurate, timely diagnoses outweigh the potential risks. There should be no hesitation to perform the most appropriate imaging study
- It is difficult to detect abruption with imaging alone

Introduction

Trauma, affects up to 7% of pregnancies and is the primary cause of non-obstetrical maternal mortality. Most pregnancy-related injuries occur in the third trimester secondary to motor vehicle crashes, domestic violence and falls. Most maternal deaths occur from head trauma and haemorrhage. The foremost cause of fetal death is maternal death. In cases of maternal shock, the fetal death rate reaches 80%. When the mother survives, the principal cause of fetal death is placental abruption. Reported fetal mortality rates from maternal blunt trauma range from 3 to 38%. Regardless of severity, all injured pregnant women should undergo fetal monitoring for 4–6 hours.

ABC of Imaging in Trauma. By Leonard J. King and David C. Wherry
Published 2010 by Blackwell Publishing

Diagnostic modalities without ionizing radiation

Fetal monitoring

Fetal heart rate (FHR) may be assessed by Doppler or ultrasound. A positive fetal heartbeat should prompt determination of gestational age (GA), as no obstetrical intervention will alter the outcome of a pre-viable fetus (<23 weeks). Regardless of gestational age, good treatment for the mother is good treatment for the fetus, as the fetus does not tolerate hypoxemia or hypovolemia.

Fetal distress is manifest by an abnormal FHR. Continuous electronic fetal monitoring is the most sensitive modality for diagnosing placental abruption. A diagnosis of abruption warrants immediate delivery as fetal mortality approaches 75%. Most placental abruptions occur within 4 hours of injury and no supporting evidence exists for monitoring beyond 24 hours.

Ultrasound

Ultrasound can safely determine FHR, GA and amniotic fluid index. Ultrasound is ideal to evaluate fetal wellbeing and placental location. Sonography may diagnose haemorrhagic amniotic fluid, uterine rupture with herniation of amniotic sac or fetal parts, or placental abruption by demonstrating retroplacental haematoma (Figure 12.1). Sensitivity for diagnosis of placental abruption is poor, however, missing 50–80% of cases.

Abdominal sonography can also be a useful test to detect the presence of haemoperitoneum in the haemodynamically unstable trauma patient. However, ultrasound becomes more technically difficult in advanced pregnancy and also fails to confidently diagnose many non-uterine injuries.

Magnetic resonance imaging (MRI)

MRI benefits from excellent soft tissue contrast and lack of ionizing radiation. In the stable patient, neurologic injuries can be well evaluated, though the use of contrast materials in the pregnant patient is not recommended. MRI may be of limited value in the third trimester due to fetal motion degrading the study. In the multiply injured trauma patient, MRI can be unsuitable, as exams times are lengthy with restricted patient access and monitoring.

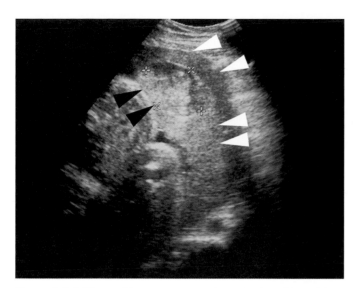

Figure 12.1 A 30-year-old pregnant woman (gestational age 30 weeks) following a motor vehicle crash. Transverse ultrasound image of gravid uterus shows placenta (white arrowheads) with associated heterogeneous haematoma (black arrowheads). Arrows indicate myometrium. (Reprinted with permission from Brown MA et al. Journal of Ultrasound Medicine 2005; **24**: 175–181)

Diagnostic modalities with ionizing radiation

Diagnostic procedures using ionizing radiation require evaluation of the risks and benefits. Although the risk from diagnostic radiation to the fetus is low, the developing fetus is more sensitive than the adult to ionizing radiation. Spontaneous abortion, small head size, poor growth, mental retardation, malformation and increased incidence of future cancers are adverse effects seen with extremely large radiation doses to the fetus. The fetus is most sensitive to deleterious effects in the first trimester, particularly exposures before 8 weeks GA. The uterus and fetus may be shielded for many radiographic studies, although some exposure can still occur due to internal scatter.

Adverse radiation effects to the fetus are improbable at doses less than 50–100 mGy. Beyond 15 weeks GA the fetus is unlikely to be affected by diagnostic levels of radiation.

Protecting the mother and unborn child are priorities, and fetal wellbeing depends on maternal wellbeing. If the mother's life is at risk and clear indications for an imaging study exist, there should be no hesitation to do the study. Moreover, if the indicated study requires direct fetal exposure, the examination should not be delayed or denied, but performed properly without hesitation. The International Commission on Radiological Protection (ICRP), National Council on Radiation Protection (NCRP), American College of Radiology (ACR), American Collage of Surgeons (ACS) and the American College of Obstetrics and Gynecology (ACOG) support these statements.

Radiography

Radiographic imaging remote from the fetus with proper collimation does not deposit significant dose (scatter only) to the con-ceptus and can be safely performed at any time during pregnancy. Unnecessary or duplicate examinations should be avoided.

Angiography

Angiographic exposures are based on fluoroscopic time, number of vessels evaluated and patient thickness. Angiography with embolization is an excellent means of controlling active haemorrhage and pseudoaneurysms, especially from bleeding pelvic vessels. Fluoroscopic exposures range from 20 to 100 mGy/min.

Computed tomography (CT)

CT remains the most sensitive, specific, accurate and cost-effective diagnostic modality to evaluate the stable trauma patient. CT is fast, non-invasive and widely available. Just as CT is able to diagnose injuries in the multiply injured non-pregnant patient, Lowdermilk et al. (1999) have shown CT to be effective in the pregnant trauma patient.

Direct fetal exposure from a pelvic CT examination approximates 25–35 mGy. The actual dose varies with patient thickness, fetal depth within the mother and CT parameters including pitch, tube current (mA) and tube voltage (kVp). Efforts should be sought to decrease doses to as low as reasonably achievable. Although no controlled human studies of intravenous contrast material safety have been performed, data from animal studies show no teratogenic or mutagenic effects.

CT imaging findings

Normal pregnancy
First trimester
The first CT signs of an intrauterine gestation are a bulging ovoid lumen within a mildly enlarged uterus (Figure 12.2). The uterine fundus grows 1 cm/week, and by 12 weeks GA, the bladder is displaced out of the bony confines of the pelvis and becomes susceptible to direct trauma.

Second trimester
The uterine fundus reaches the umbilicus at 20 weeks GA. Fetal parts are evident by the late first or early second trimester. Discrete skeletal structures are readily seen by the end of the second trimester. Placental cotyledons demonstrate a repeating pattern of hyperdense rings with lower central attenuation. Engorged vessels deep to the placenta identify its insertion site (Figure 12.3).

Third trimester
By the third trimester the uterus compresses the upper maternal abdominal organs against the ribs and the diaphragm. Fetal stomach and bladder are seen as fluid-filled structures. A lack of appreciable fetal organ enhancement is normal as only a small amount of intravenous contrast material crosses the placenta (Figures 12.4a and 12.4b).

Maternal changes with pregnancy
As maternal blood volume increases with pregnancy, ovarian vein enlargement is seen, approaching the size of the inferior vena cava (IVC). The most marked structural change is hydronephrosis of

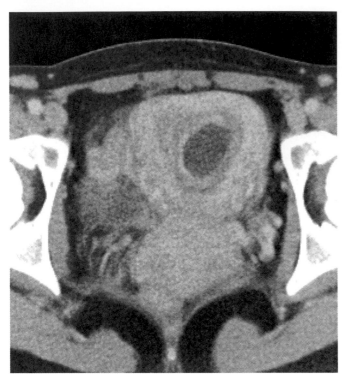

Figure 12.2 A 21-year-old pregnant woman (gestational age 6 weeks) with abdominal pain and fever. Contrast-enhanced CT shows bulging gestational sac in mildly enlarged uterus of normal first trimester. (Reprinted with permission from Bernstein MP. 2008 ARRS Categorical Course: State-of-the-Art Emergency and Trauma Radiology 2008.)

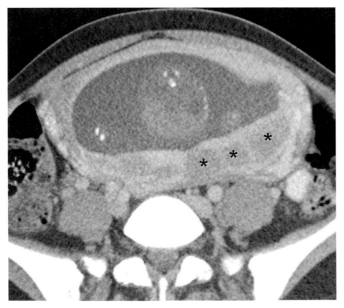

Figure 12.3 A 24-year-old pregnant woman (gestational age 14 weeks) with abdominal pain. Contrast-enhanced CT shows placental cotyledons (asterisks) and peripherally engorged vessels of normal second trimester.

pregnancy (Figure 12.4c). Diastasis of the pubic symphysis and sacroiliac joints may be seen in late pregnancy.

Patterns of injury
Maternal
The pregnant patient is more susceptible to genitourinary injuries in the setting of a dilated collecting system and elevated bladder. Pelvic ligament laxity places the bony pelvis at risk of injury, and increased pelvic blood flow predisposes to fetomaternal haemorrhage. Consequently, pelvic fractures are the most common injury leading to fetal demise (Figure 12.5).

Injuries to the head, spine, chest, torso and extremities of non-pregnant patients similarly occur in pregnant trauma patients. Severe maternal head injury is strongly associated with fetal loss. Compression of the liver and spleen against the costal margins by the gravid uterus increase the risk of hepatic and splenic injuries.

No significant differences in morbidity were noted between ruptures of a scarred (prior caesarian section) or unscarred uterus.

Placental/uterine
Sudden deceleration may result in shearing of the relatively rigid placenta from the more elastic uterus, causing placental abruption. Abruption of more than 50% of the placental interface leads to fetal death. On CT, placental abruption or infarction can be seen as regions of placental non-enhancement, and are the most common uteroplacental injuries (Figures 12.5 and 12.6). CT may also identify uterine lacerations and contusions. Uterine rupture is an ominous sign (see Box 12.1). Fetal expulsion into the maternal peritoneum from uterine rupture has been reported (Figure 12.7).

Penetrating abdominal trauma to the pregnant patient is strongly associated with direct fetal injury by the middle of the second trimester, often secondarily protecting maternal organs from injury.

Fetal
Gestational age correlates directly with fetal outcome; lower gestational age correlates significantly with fetal demise. Direct observation of fetal injuries is exceptional, but injuries such as fetal skull fractures or intracranial hemorrhage may be demonstrated (Figure 12.8).

Conclusion

A multidisciplinary team approach provides the best chance for survival for the traumatized pregnant woman and her unborn child. Efforts are focused on treating maternal injuries, as no fetal survival can occur without maternal survival. Fetal death most often follows maternal death. When the mother survives, fetal loss most commonly results from placental abruption. Lower gestational age significantly correlates with fetal demise. Major and minor trauma warrant continuous fetoplacental monitoring. Ultrasound and CT offer complementary roles in assessing fetal and maternal injuries respectively. Diagnostic radiation doses and risks are low, and the benefits of accurate, timely diagnoses outweigh the potential risks of screening CT. There should be no hesitation to perform the most appropriate study to aid in triage and management of trauma in pregnancy.

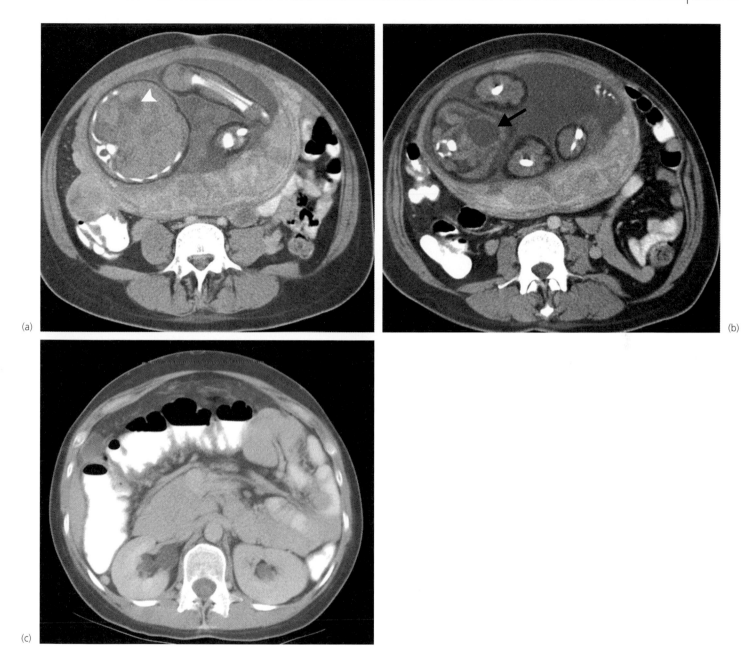

(a)

(b)

(c)

Figure 12.4 A 26-year-old pregnant woman (gestational age 33 weeks) with abdominal pain. Contrast-enhanced CT through gravid uterus shows (a) fluid-filled fetal stomach (white arrowhead) and (b) bladder (black arrow). (c) A 32-year-old pregnant woman (gestational age 32 weeks) with right lower quadrant abdominal pain. Contrast-enhanced CT shows maternal hydronephrosis of pregnancy in normal third trimester.

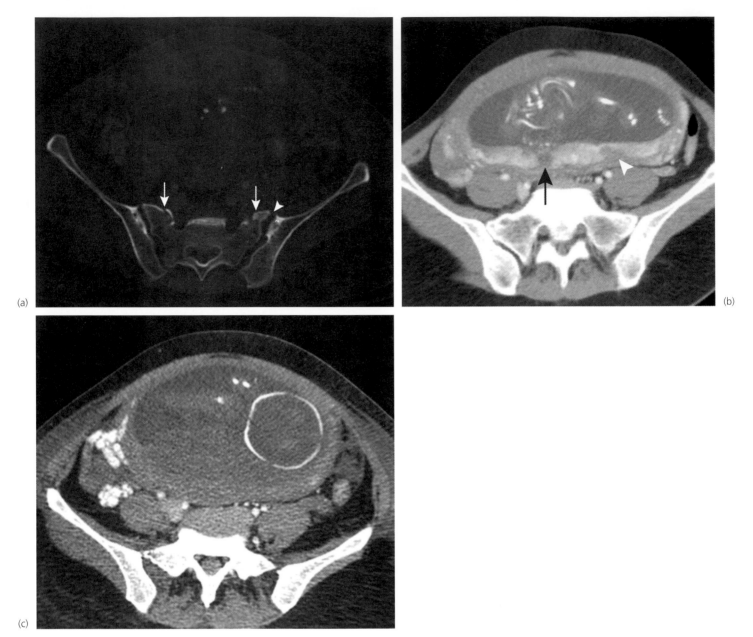

(a)

(b)

(c)

Figure 12.5 A 34-year-old pregnant woman (gestational age 22 weeks) with injuries sustained as pedestrian struck by motor vehicle. (a) Contrast-enhanced CT through pelvis shows bilateral sacral alar fractures (arrows) and diastasis of the left sacroiliac joint (arrowhead). (b) Contrast-enhanced CT through gravid uterus shows foci of partial (white arrowhead) and full-thickness (black arrow) placental non-enhancement, consistent with abruption. (c) Follow-up contrast-enhanced CT through gravid uterus 5 days after admission shows complete lack of placental enhancement consistent with total infarction. The fetus did not survive.

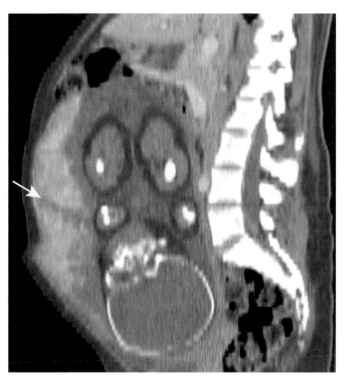

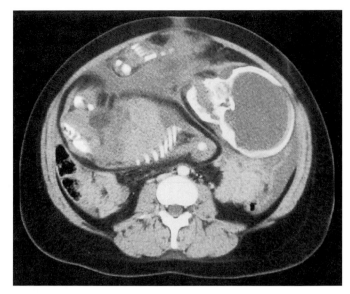

Figure 12.6 A 33-year-old pregnant woman (gestational age 36 weeks) with injuries sustained as a passenger in a motor vehicle collisioin. Contrast-enhanced sagittal CT reformation through gravid uterus shows placental perfusion defect (arrow).

Figure 12.7 A 25-year-old pregnant woman (gestational age 39 weeks) with injuries sustained as the driver in a motor vehicle collision with airbag deployment. Contrast-enhanced CT through the abdomen shows free-floating fetus with no surrounding uterus. Exploratory laparotomy confirmed uterine rupture and fetal demise. The patient survived and was discharged on postoperative day 5. (Reprinted with permission from Fusco A et al. *Journal of Trauma* 2001; **51**: 1192–1194.)

Box 12.1 **Organ injury scale for the pregnant uterus**

Grade*	Injury description
I	Contusion/haematoma (without placental abruption)
II	Superficial laceration (≤1 cm) *or* partial placental abruption <25%
III	Deep laceration (>1 cm) in second or third trimester *or* placental abruption >25% but <50%
IV	Laceration involving uterine artery *or* deep laceration (>1 cm) with > 0% placental abruption
V	Uterine rupture *or* complete placental abruption

*Advance one grade for multiple injuries up to grade III. (Moore EE et al. 1995)

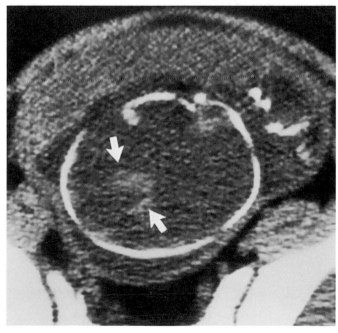

Figure 12.8 Fetal injury in a pregnant patient after trauma. Contrast-enhanced CT through gravid uterus shows fetal skull fracture and intraventricular haemorrhage (arrows). (Reprinted with permission from Goldman MA & Wagner LK. *Radiographics* 1999; **19**: 1349–1357.)

References

Lowdermilk C, Gavant ML, Qaisi W *et al*. Screening helical CT for evaluation of blunt traumatic injury in the pregnant patient. *Radiographics* 1999; **19**: S243–255.

Moore EE *et al*. Organ injury scaling. Part VI. Extrahepatic biliary, esophagus, stomach, vulva, vagina, uterus (nonpregnant), uterus (pregnant), fallopian tube, and ovary. *Journal of Trauma* 1995; **39**: 1069–1070.

Further reading

Committee on Obstetric Practice. Guidelines for diagnostic imaging during pregnancy: ACOG Committee opinion no. 299, September 2004 (replaces no. 158, September 1995). *Obstetrics and Gynecology* 2004; **104**: 647–651.

Goldman SM & Wagner LK. Radiologic ABCs of maternal and fetal survival after trauma: when minutes may count. *Radiographics* 1999; **19**: 1349–1357.

International Commission on Radiological Protection. Pregnancy and medical radiation. *Annals of the ICRP* 2000; **30**: 1–43.

Mattox KL & Goetzl L. Trauma in pregnancy. *Critical Care Medicine* 2005; **33**: S385–389.

CHAPTER 13

Bullets, Bombs and Ballistics

Peter K. Ellis[1], Iain Gibb[2] and James Ryan[3]

[1]Royal Victoria Hospital, Belfast, Northern Ireland, UK
[2]Royal Hospital Haslar, Gosport, Hampshire, UK
[3]University College London and St George's University of London, London, UK *and* Uniformed Services University of the Health Sciences, Bethesda, MD, USA

OVERVIEW

- The nature of firearms and their projectiles
- Ballistics and the factors that determine the nature of injury from gunshot wounds
- Imaging of gunshot wounds
- The nature of bomb blasts and the injuries that can occur
- The imaging of blast-related injuries

Ballistics

To understand the mechanisms of gunshot injuries it is helpful to appreciate the nature of firearms and projectiles. Ballistics is the science of the travel of a projectile in flight, including its behaviour during wounding. The combination of internal, external and terminal (wound) ballistics determines the nature of the resulting injuries that a projectile will incur.

Internal ballistics

Internal ballistics concerns the projectile within the gun. A bullet is held within a cartridge case, which contains a flammable propellant (charge) with a primer at its base. The firing pin strikes the primer igniting the charge, which rapidly expands, propelling the bullet from the cartridge case along the barrel of the gun (Figure 13.1). A larger charge can be used in rifle cartridges as the bullet chamber can withstand greater pressures. The long barrel of a rifle also allows more time for bullet acceleration and thus rifle bullets tend to travel at a faster velocity than bullets fired from handguns. Gun barrels contain spiral ridges or grooves (rifling), which cause a bullet to spin around its long axis giving it a degree of stability in the air.

ABC of Imaging in Trauma. By Leonard J. King and David C. Wherry
Published 2010 by Blackwell Publishing

External ballistics

External ballistics describes the behaviour of the projectile in flight. Bullets travel in a parabolic trajectory rather than in a straight line and are subject to a variety of rotational forces in their passage through air. Their behaviour is determined by a complex interaction of variables, including the ballistic coefficient of the bullet, muzzle velocity and external forces, including wind plus ambient air density. The ideal bullet would be a long, heavy needle; however, such an entity would not disperse much kinetic energy within the target. A bullet must have sufficient mass to penetrate and impart kinetic energy to the target and thus cause wounding. The range of shot, stability, velocity and consistency of a bullet determine the nature of impact.

Terminal ballistics

Terminal ballistics describes the behaviour of a projectile when it hits a target, and determines the resulting injuries and thus the imaging appearances. Low-velocity bullets (such as those from handguns) do most of their damage by crushing and lacerating tissue in the path of the missile. A low-velocity round fired at long range may remain within the superficial tissues thereby causing minimal injury.

Higher-velocity bullets cause injury by cavitation and shock waves. The bullet itself forms a permanent cavity and there is an additional temporary cavity formed by continuing movement of the tissue in the wake of the bullet, with the potential for more extensive injury (Figure 13.2). Tissues with higher specific gravities and lower elasticity will incur greater damage. Thus lung tissue is damaged less than solid organs such as brain and liver. Fluid-filled organs are susceptible to the pressure waves generated. Bones may fracture or cause fragmentation of the bullet, with secondary projectiles each producing additional wounds (Figures 13.3a and 13.3b).

Imaging of gunshot wounds

Bullet design is important in the assessment of gunshot wounds (GSWs). Most bullets are made of lead and may be encased in a metal jacket to protect the lead from deformity and melting,

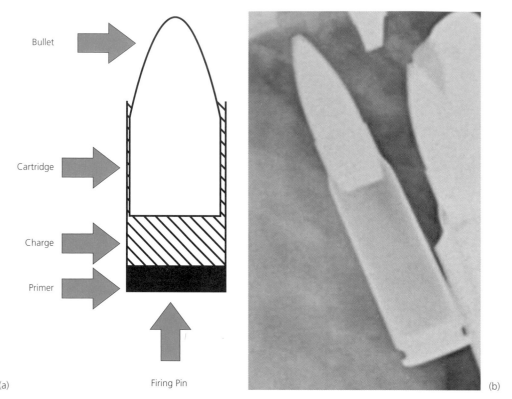

Bullet

Cartridge

Charge

Primer

(a)   Firing Pin   (b)

Figure 13.1 (a) Diagrammatic representation of a bullet. (b) Radiograph of an unused high velocity round complete with casing demonstrating the component parts.

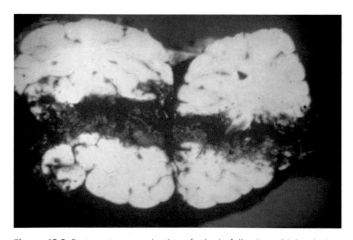

Figure 13.2 Post-mortem examination of a brain following a high-velocity bullet wound that traversed the cranium. Note the extent of injury is considerably more than the diameter of a bullet due to cavitation.

particularly with high-velocity weapons. A copper jacket is most frequently used and the encased bullet is said to have a "full metal jacket". Some bullets leave lead exposed at the tip (semi-jacketed), which deforms on impact forming a mushroom shape. This causes the bullet to decelerate faster, thus delivering more energy and increasing tissue damage. Hollow-point bullets have a similar effect.

When a bullet strikes the target it tends to tumble around its short axis and, if the wound track is of sufficient length, may rotate through 180 degrees and end up pointing backwards towards the entry point (Figure 13.4). A fully jacketed rifle bullet may pass straight through a target; however, a low-velocity lead round will often remain within the injured tissue and demonstrate evidence of deformity. This can be useful in the assessment of patient safety for magnetic resonance imaging (MRI). Shotgun pellets made of lead will demonstrate deformity, whereas steel shotgun pellets, which are less MRI safe, will not.

Bones affect the behaviour of bullets by altering their course on impact and causing fragmentation. The evaluation of bony injuries on plain radiographs can help to determine the direction of travel of the projectile. Bevelling of the bone and a cone of bullet fragmentation are useful pointers in this regard (Figure 13.5). The apex of the cone points towards the entry site.

If plain radiographs are used to assess bullet injuries, views should be obtained in two orthogonal projections. This will allow some degree of localization of fragments. A metal marker such as a paper clip placed at the entry site can also help to determine the internal pathway of the bullet, giving a guide to the tissues that are likely to have been injured (Figure 13.6).

Computed tomography (CT) can be extremely useful for demonstrating bullet fragments (despite the artefact that may occur) and wound tracts, which may be outlined by air, haemorrhage, bullet fragments, bone fragments or external foreign bodies such

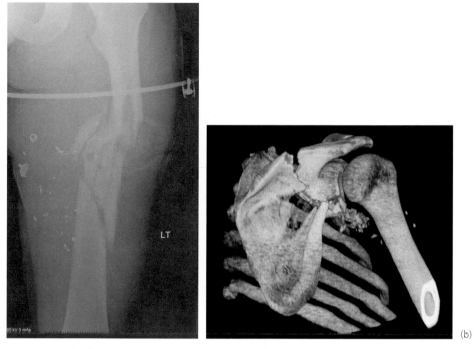

(a)

(b)

Figure 13.3 (a) Anteroposterior radiograph of a high-velocity gunshot wound to the left thigh demonstrating a comminuted fracture and extensive bullet fragmentation. (b) 3D volume-rendered CT scan of the right shoulder demonstrating a comminuted fracture of the scapula due to a high-velocity gunshot wound.

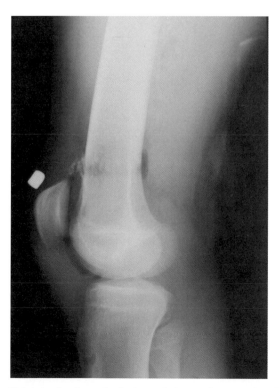

Figure 13.4 Lateral radiograph of a low-velocity gunshot wound to the leg with a posterior entry wound above the popliteal fossa. The intact bullet remains within the soft tissues and has rotated through almost 180° to face the entry point. Air partially outlines the bullet tract and there is air within the knee joint. There is also some bevelling of the distal femur, which points away from the entry site.

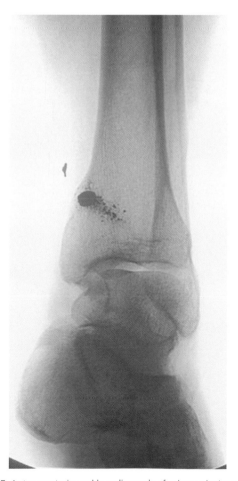

Figure 13.5 Anteroposterior ankle radiograph of a low-velocity gunshot wound to the left ankle from a superomedial direction. There is relatively little bone damage but there is a cone of bullet fragmentation, the apex of which points towards the entry point.

as clothing (Figure 13.7). The entry wound and the exit wound, if present, can be difficult to determine with accuracy; however, secondary signs such as bone bevelling and a cone of bone fragmentation along the direction of the bullet path may be useful. CT is particularly useful in abdominal injuries for demonstrating organ lacerations and contrast extravasation, indicating active bleeding

(Figure 13.8). Vascular injuries can also be detected, prompting angiography (Figure 13.9) and possibly operative or endovascular management.

Endovascular treatment options include the use of coils to occlude a non-essential artery (Figure 13.10), balloon occlusion to prevent bleeding while a patient is transferred to the operating

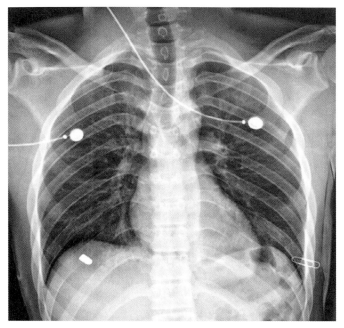

Figure 13.6 Chest radiograph demonstrating a thoracic gunshot wound. The paper clip denotes the entry wound in the lower left hemithorax remote from the in situ bullet, which is projected just below the right hemidiaphragm.

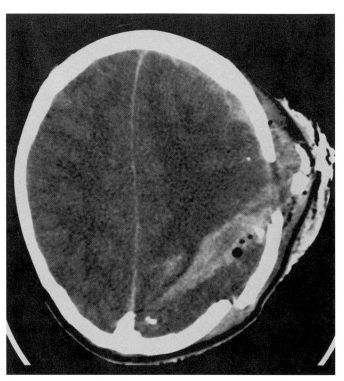

Figure 13.7 CT scan of brain following a gunshot wound demonstrates a soft tissue tract with air, blood and bony fragments.

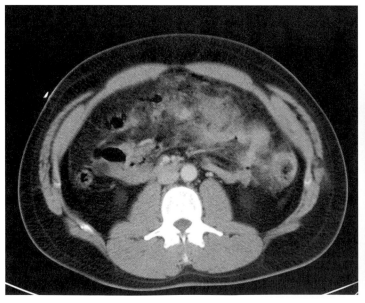

(a)

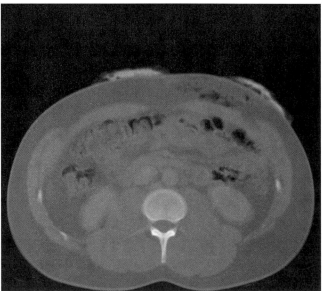

(b)

Figure 13.8 Abdominal CT scans in two different patients with gunshot wounds. (a) A transabdominal wound that has breached the peritoneal cavity with bowel and mesenteric injury. (b) A superficial wound traversing only the subcutaneous fat layer with no breach of the peritoneal cavity or major intra-abdominal injury.

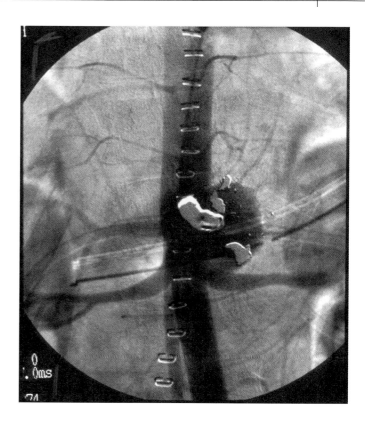

Figure 13.9 Aortic angiogram demonstrating pseudoaneurysm of the abdominal aorta. Bullet fragments overlie the pseudoaneurysm and there is occlusion of the splenic artery.

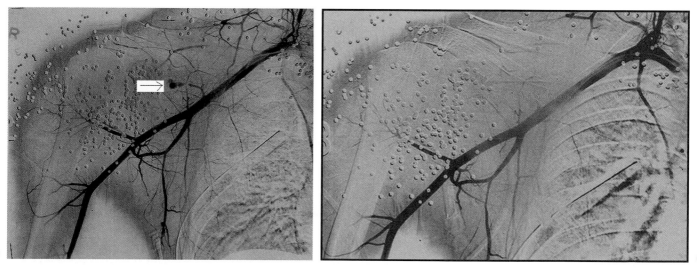

(a)   (b)

Figure 13.10 (a) Gunshot wound to the shoulder with active extravasation noted from a small superior branch of the axillary artery (arrow). (b) A micro-catheter was placed within the branch from a transfemoral approach and a single coil used to occlude the vessel with good effect.

theatre, covered stent placement (although caution may be required where there is an open, contaminated wound) and endovascular removal of intravascular bullet fragments or pellets (Figure 13.11).

In riot control situations, rubber bullets and plastic baton rounds (Figure 13.12a) may be used. These are large projectiles that travel at relatively low velocities and cause injury by crushing. They are designed to be fired at a particular range (approximately 30 metres); however, this is often difficult to achieve in a riot situation and significant injuries and even death can occur as a result of their use (Figure 13.12b).

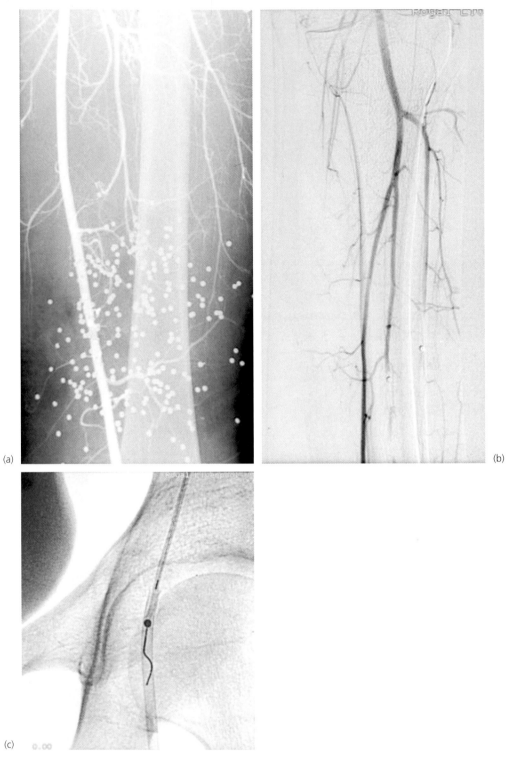

(a)

(b)

(c) 0.00

Figure 13.11 (a) Gunshot wound to the thigh with multiple small pellets (birdshot). The femoral artery does not appear injured. (b) Several pellets have embolized distally in the calf, occluding the peroneal and anterior tibial arteries. (c) The pellets were removed percutaneously via an antegrade common femoral approach using a small snare. (Images courtesy of Dr Richard Edwards. Previously published in *Clinical Radiology* 1996; **51**: 140–143.)

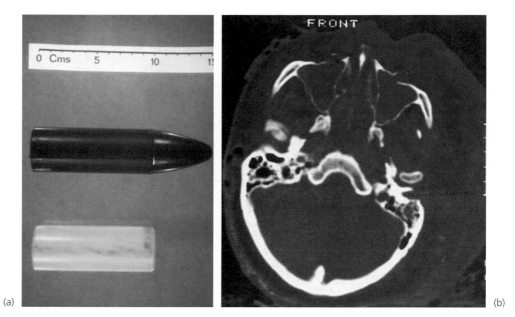

Figure 13.12 (a) Rubber bullet (top) and a plastic baton round (bottom). The scale is in centimetres. (b) CT scan demonstrating extensive soft tissue injuries and left-sided maxillary fracture as a result of a plastic baton round.

Imaging of blast injuries

Blast injuries may result from domestic or industrial accidents, such as gas explosions, or as a result of military action and terrorist bombings.

When a bomb is detonated it can produce injury by several discrete mechanisms (Box 13.1). There is an initial shock wave, which travels at very high velocity and may be deflected around corners and off solid surfaces, which can augment the potential for injury. This shock wave has the potential to cause primary injury, particularly at air/fluid interfaces, notably in the lung. Pulmonary barotrauma is the most common fatal primary blast injury. The shock wave causes injury to pulmonary capillary/alveolar interfaces, resulting in contusion, thrombosis, haemorrhagic contamination of the alveoli and disseminated intravascular coagulation. Haemothorax, pneumothorax, bronchopleural fistulae and rib fractures may also occur. Initial chest radiographs may be relatively normal; however, patients with pulmonary barotrauma rapidly develop pulmonary infiltrates similar to pulmonary contusion and adult respiratory distress syndrome (Figure 13.13). The blast wave may cause acute gas embolism, resulting in occlusion of blood vessels, particularly affecting the brain and spinal cord. The primary blast wave can also cause spinal and limb fractures, although these are more likely to be caused by projectiles or whole body displacement.

The blast wind then follows; it travels at lower velocity than the shock wave but with considerably more energy due to expanding gases. It is not symmetrical and will travel in a direction determined by the manufacture of the bomb and the environment in which it is placed. This blast wind will propel fragments, such as glass from fragmented windows and other components of buildings or vehicles, resulting in penetrating injury, which is the most common clinical presentation following exposure to blast. This is referred to as secondary injury and can also occur as a result of deliberately

> **Box 13.1 Definition of primary, secondary, tertiary and quaternary blast-related injury**
>
> ***Primary injury*** – due to blast shock wave travelling at greater than speed of sound, e.g. lungs and tympanic membranes
> ***Secondary injury*** – fragments generated in the blast environment (primary from the casing or secondary from the environment)
> ***Tertiary injury*** – displacement by the blast winds result in, for example, traumatic amputation
> ***Quaternary injury*** – burns, crush injuries, smoke inhalation, etc., and post-traumatic stress syndromes

placed nails or other metallic objects around the bomb casing (Figure 13.14). With blasts in open spaces, injuries due to flying objects can occur up to several kilometres away from the seat of the explosion. Penetrating fragments may result in injury to the brain, chest or abdominal organs. Imaging with CT can be useful to determine the position, effect and necessity for removal of fragments. The blast wind can also result in whole body displacement and disruption of the environment, which may produce severe injury, including traumatic amputation (Figure 13.15). Injuries caused by displacement are referred to as tertiary injuries.

A fireball typically occurs when a device explodes and may singe exposed skin. However, most significant burns occur as a result of secondary fires and can be severe. Burns are classified as quaternary injury.

Crush injuries may occur as a result of falling masonry and other displaced heavy objects. Morbidity or mortality can also occur due to radiation exposure or the presence of toxic dust or gas (bomb casings may be coated with toxins like cyanide). Psychological effects are common, may affect those even some distance from the blast site and are often underestimated.

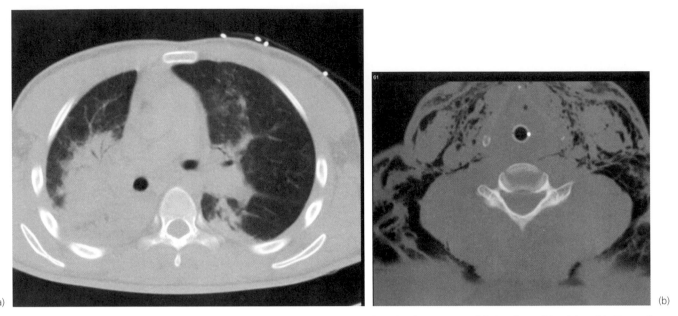

(a)

(b)

Figure 13.13 (a) Chest CT scan following an explosion in an enclosed space. There is bilateral pulmonary consolidation due to blast injury. (b) CT scan from a different patient with extensive surgical emphysema due to blast injury.

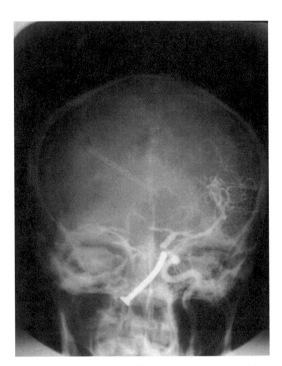

Figure 13.14 Anteroposterior view (from a conventional carotid arteriogram) taken of a victim of a blast where the bomb casing was coated with nails. Notice the nail is causing calibre change at the distal internal carotid artery on the left side.

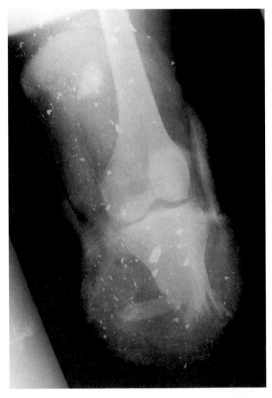

Figure 13.15 Anteroposterior radiograph of the lower leg demonstrating a traumatic amputation due to blast injury from an improvised explosive device.

Explosions within a confined space are more likely to result in severe blast loading and result in primary blast injury to lungs, heart and the brain. Death or severe injuries such as dismemberment are common in a blast in a confined space. Bowel injuries are most likely to occur with underwater explosions.

The tympanic membranes are particularly susceptible to blast injury. Rupture of the tympanic membrane is commonly seen and may be treated conservatively. Tympanic injury is a rough marker for the presence of more widespread exposure to blast; however, the absence of injury does not allow exclusion of other blast-related injuries.

Imaging of blast injuries principally concerns the detection of pressure injuries such as pulmonary barotrauma and fragment wounds. Plain radiographs can be useful for demonstration of pulmonary, spinal and limb injuries, as well as the presence of penetrating fragments. CT will often provide additional information about the presence and severity of organ or vascular injury and the exact location of retained fragments, but should not delay damage limitation surgery in unstable patients who require immediate intervention. Suspected vascular injuries may also be assessed with angiography and in some cases can be treated by endovascular means.

Further references

Barnett DJ, Parker CL, Blogett DW *et al.* Understanding radiological and nuclear terrorism as public health threats: preparedness and response oerspectives. *Journal of Nuclear Medicine* 2006; **47**: 1653–1661.

Hare SS, Goddard I, Ward P *et al.* The radiological management of bomb blast injury. *Clinical Radiology* 2007; **62**: 1–9.

Sosna J, Tamar S, Dorith S *et al.* Facing the new threats of terrorism: radiologists' perspectives based on experience in Israel. *Radiology* 2005; **237**: 28–36.

Swan KG & Swan RC. Principles of ballistics applicable to the treatment of gunshot wounds. *Surgical Clinics of North America* 1991; **71**: 221–239.

Wilson AJ. Gunshot injuries: what does a radiologist need to know? *Radiographics* 1999; **19**: 1358–1368.

CHAPTER 14

Imaging of Major Incidents and Mass Casualty Situations

James H. Street¹, Christopher Burns², Xzabia Caliste¹, Mark W. Bowyer³ and Leonard J. King⁴

¹Washington Hospital Center, Washington, DC, USA
²National Naval Medical Center, Bethesda, MD, USA
³Uniformed Services University of the Health Sciences, Bethesda, MD, USA
⁴Southampton University Hospitals NHS Trust, Southampton, Hampshire, UK

OVERVIEW

- In mass casualty events the number of patients can overwhelm a medical facility
- Accurate triage is important to determine treatment priorities
- Imaging can assist in triaging patients' needs for treatment
- Plain radiographs are commonly utilized in this setting
- Ultrasound is helpful for screening multiple casualties but has diagnostic limitations
- Computed tomography should be initially reserved for casualties with the greatest need
- New, faster radiographic imaging systems including the Lodox Statscan allow faster image acquisition and can increase patient throughput

---

Mass casualty incident

During mass casualty incidents the number of ill or injured patients exceeds the available healthcare resources. Such incidents can be the result of military action, acts of terrorism, catastrophic events such as a train crash or natural disasters such as an earthquake. This differs from a multiple casualty event in which several injured patients are received by a medical facility at the same time.

During mass casualty incidents, and to a lesser extent multiple casualty incidents, the presence of a large number of casualties may lower the quality of care given to individual patients due to limitations in time, personnel, equipment and medical supplies. Optimal care of patients in these circumstances requires well-thought-out and practised disaster plans with the goal of providing a level of care that approximates the care given to similar patients under normal conditions. During mass casualty events it is important to

rapidly identify patients with life-threatening, but survivable, injuries, who require immediate intervention. This is best accomplished by effective triage in which imaging modalities can have a limited but useful role.

Triage

Triage is an attempt to impose order during chaos and make an initially overwhelming situation manageable. Triage is a dynamic process of sorting casualties to identify the treatment priorities given the limitations of the situation and available resources. Traditional categories of triage are:

- immediate – requiring immediate intervention to save life
- delayed – require intervention but general status permits delay
- minimal – minor injuries
- expectant – casualties whose wounds are so extensive that they are unlikely to survive even with maximal treatment.

Triage decisions need to be made rapidly by assessing factors such as initial vital signs, the pattern of injury and response to the initial intervention. Imaging modalities that can be performed quickly and have a likelihood of helping triage patients are a useful adjunct to the management of multiple or mass casualty events.

Plain radiography in mass casualty events

Standard radiography retains an important role in the management of multiple or mass casualties (Figure 14.1). The most important radiographs (and probably the only) to obtain in the initial phase of multiple casualty management are chest and pelvic films, as abnormal findings on these images will often mandate immediate intervention. In true mass casualty situations, radiography should initially be limited to those patients in whom clinical evaluation suggests that they would be most likely to benefit.

Modern digital radiography equipment has significantly reduced image processing time and has greater exposure latitude compared to conventional radiography. This reduces image acquisition time and repeat exposures, allowing increased patient throughput.

ABC of Imaging in Trauma. By Leonard J. King and David C. Wherry
Published 2010 by Blackwell Publishing

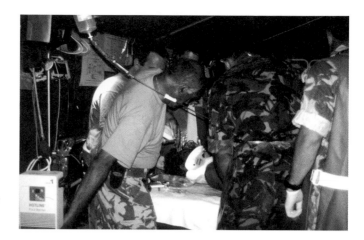

Figure 14.1 A military radiographer (far right) prepares to take portable radiographs of a male patient during a multiple casualty situation in a tented field hospital.

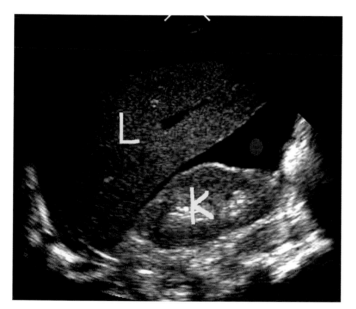

Figure 14.2 An ultrasound image of the right upper quadrant showing free fluid (red dot) between the kidney (K) and the liver (L).

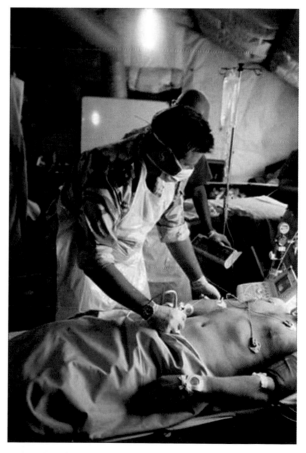

Figure 14.3 A military surgeon using a portable ultrasound machine to perform a FAST exam on a patient with a blunt abdominal trauma in a field hospital.

Ultrasound application in mass casualty events

Ultrasound has several potential advantages as a triage tool in mass casualty events, being quick, non-invasive and relatively simple to perform. In many studies, the focused assessment with sonography for trauma (FAST) exam has been shown to be accurate, sensitive and specific for the demonstration of free fluid. The FAST exam can be performed rapidly (usually in less than 2–4 minutes) to screen trauma patients for pericardial, pleural or intra-abdominal fluid (Figure 14.2). The technique can be carried out by non-radiologists with limited training, making it particularly useful in austere circumstances where there is limited imaging support. With appropriate training and experience, ultrasound can also be used to diagnose pneumothorax and some fractures, and it lends itself well to serial examinations without exposure to ionizing radiation. Robust handheld units make this technology highly portable and have proved to be a very useful tool in the deployed military setting (Figure 14.3) where environmental conditions can be hostile and power supplies unpredictable.

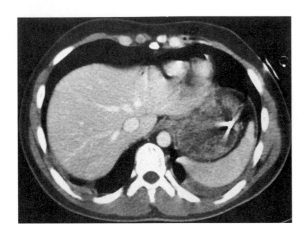

Figure 14.4 A male casualty with a blast injury from an improvised explosive device who had multiple seemingly superficial wounds on the abdominal wall. Abdominal CT scan demonstrates a metallic fragment that had perforated the patient's stomach.

There are several reports of the successful use of ultrasound during mass casualty situations, including earthquakes in Armenia and Turkey as well as in several military theatres of operations. However, it is important to recognize the limitations of ultrasound in excluding significant injury particularly in the retroperitoneum.

The role of computed tomography in mass casualty events

While computed tomography (CT) is the imaging modality of choice for assessing victims of major trauma, its routine use in mass casualty situations cannot be advocated given the time required to acquire images and the need to transport patients. The advent of multi-detector CT scanners has reduced image acquisition time, particularly for whole-body imaging; however, patient transfers on and off the scanner plus the set-up and planning phase of scanning can still take several minutes. Image post-processing, such as producing multiplaner refomats of the spine or pelvis, and diagnostic review of more than a thousand images by the supervising radiologist also takes time particularly with complex cases. Thus achieving a throughput of more than around four patients per scanner per hour for whole-body CT is difficult even with experienced staff. CT should therefore be limited in mass casualty situations to the most essential cases, including those with serious head injuries in whom CT can help to determine which patients have a potentially salvageable injury and would benefit from surgery. In multiple casualty situations CT may play a more important role as dictated by local resources, particularly if multiple scanners and personnel are available. Military combat support hospitals have also found rapid access to CT scanning to be useful in screening victims of blast injury with multiple penetrating wounds (Figure 14.4).

Lodox statscan low-dose digital radiography system and its potential use for mass casualties

The Lodox Statscan (Benmore, South Africa) is a flexible-format, low-dose digital radiography system used for rapid medical diagnoses in trauma centres and emergency departments. The original Statscan system was designed for use in the South African mining industry, to search for hidden diamonds in the clothes and body cavities of mine workers. This need to frequently monitor a large population required a time-efficient system with excellent image quality and radiation levels low enough to be used on a daily basis. It became readily apparent that the bones of the workers were also clearly imaged, and the medical imaging consultants working on the project recognized its potential use in the health sciences. The system was subsequently modified for trauma and emergency medicine. After an initial trial in a South African Level 1 trauma centre the machine was approved for use and is available in a handful of trauma centres around the world.

The technique is similar to the acquisition of CT scanogram images and utilizes a C-arm mounted x-ray tube allowing acquisition of frontal, oblique and lateral views (Figure 14.5). The Statscan provides full-body anteroposterior (AP) radiographs in around 13 seconds, detecting fractures or other injuries that may not be immediately apparent on primary or secondary survey (Figures 14.6 and 14.7). While it is critical to treat the most life-threatening injuries first, according to the ABC principles, early recognition of major limb fractures can help explain clinically occult blood loss in patients with shock, and a delayed or missed secondary injury can be detrimental to the eventual patient outcome. The total-body scan can also help medical staff to determine the approximate path of a bullet or blast fragment, without the need for a montage of multiple body area radiographs (Figures 14.8 and 14.9).

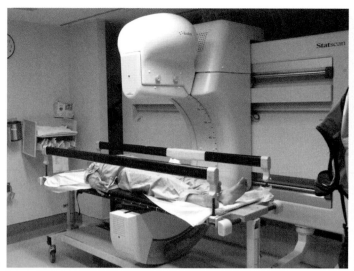
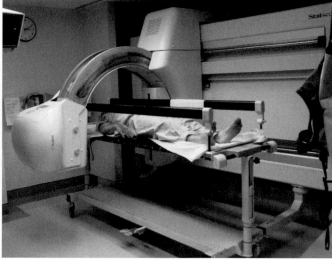

(a)

(b)

Figure 14.5 The Lodox Statscan performing (a) anteroposterior (AP) and (b) lateral total body digital radiographs.

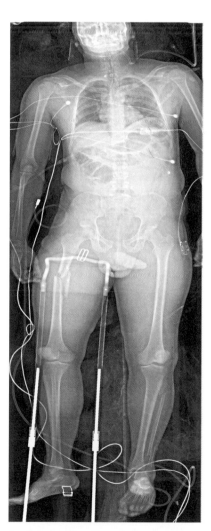

Figure 14.6 Lodox Statscan AP radiograph demonstrating satisfactory positioning of the in situ endotracheal plus nasogastric tubes, a subtle left apical pneumothorax, a metallic foreign body projected over the thoracic outlet, a right scapular fracture, an open book pelvic fracture, a right femur fracture, left fibular fractures and subluxation of the left ankle.

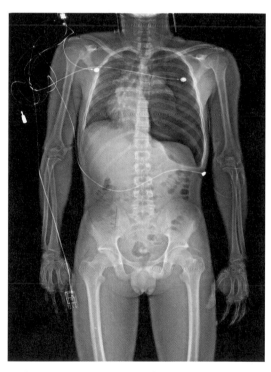

Figure 14.7 Lodox Statscan AP radiograph of a haemodynamically stable patient involved in a motor vehicle collision demonstrating a large left tension pneumothorax requiring urgent intervention.

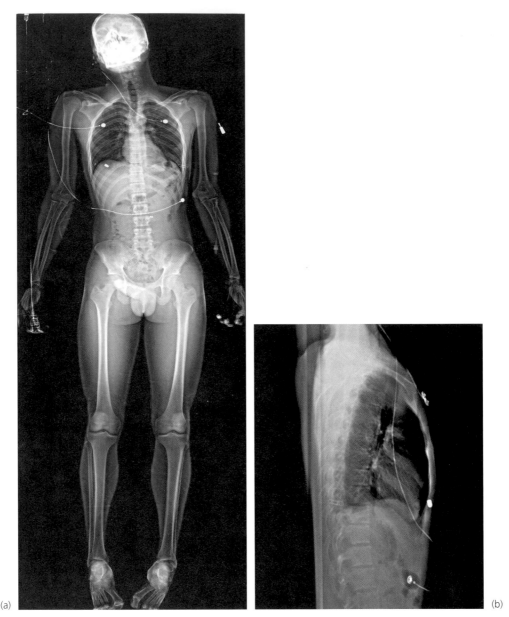

(a)   (b)

Figure 14.8 Lodox Statscan images of a casualty with a gunshot wound to the left posterolateral chest. (a) The AP image shows the entrance wound (demarcated by a paper clip) with an associated left 9th rib fracture and a retained bullet projected over the right hemidiaphragm. (b) The lateral view demonstrates that the bullet is lying anteriorly in the chest wall, indicating a probable transmediastinal tract from left posterior to right anterior.

The open design allows medical personnel to have access to critically injured patients, even during the actual scanning process. The healthcare worker can remain a short distance (4 feet) from the patient without significant radiation exposure and there is no need for a shielded room. The acquired images are in digital format and may be viewed immediately on a diagnostic viewing station or remotely across a picture archiving and communication network. Relative patient radiation doses for this technique compared to conventional radiography, vary from 72% (chest) to 2% (pelvis), with a simple average of between 6% and 25%. Imaging takes on average 3–4 minutes to obtain AP and lateral whole-body images

for each patient, compared with 8–48 minutes for conventional radiographs. The image resolution of this system is similar to conventional computed radiography (CR) systems, and detailed enough to demonstrate most significant fractures.

In most centres, the Statscan is mainly used for evaluating trauma patients who are comatose or inebriated, and patients with multiple penetrating injuries to search for retained bullets or fragments. Recent studies have shown that the use of a Lodox machine substantially reduces the time taken for resuscitation, without compromising diagnostic accuracy. In a mass casualty situation the Statscan has clear advantages over conventional radi-

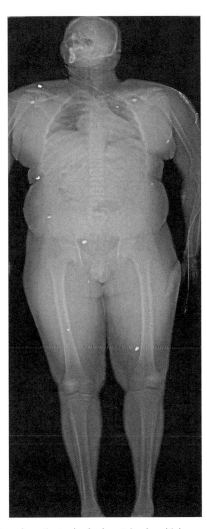

ography by providing rapid one-stop, whole-body radiographic images, improving casualty throughput and aiding the triage of multiple patients.

Further reading

Boffard KD, Goosen J, Plani F *et al.* The use of low dosage x-ray (Lodox/Statscan) in major trauma: comparison between low dose x-ray and conventional x-ray techniques. *Journal of Trauma, Injury, Infection, and Critical Care* 2006; **60**: 1175–1183.

King LJ. Ultrasound in austere and mass casualty settings. In: Brooks A, Connolly J & Chan O (eds) *Ultrasound in Emergency Care.* Blackwell, Oxford, 2004.

Ma OJ, Norvell JG & Subramanian S. Ultrasound applications in mass casualties and extreme environments. *Critical Care Medicine* 2007; **35**(5 suppl): S275–279.

Miller LA & Mirvis SE. Total-body digital radiography for trauma screening: initial experience. *Applied Radiology* 2004; **33**(8): 8–14.

Mulligan ME & Flye CW. Initial experience with Lodox Statscan imaging system for detecting injuries of the pelvis and appendicular skeleton. *Emergency Radiology* 2006; **13**(3): 129–133.

Triage. In: *Emergency War Surgery*, 3rd US revision. Borden Institute, Walter Reed Army Medical Center, Washington, DC, 2004: 3.1–3.17.

Figure 14.9 A male patient who had sustained multiple gunshot wounds. A Lodox Statscan whole-body image demonstrates multiple bullets projected over the right acromioclavicular joint, the left chest, the pelvis, right groin plus the subcutaneous tissues of the upper abdomen and posterior thighs.

Index

ABC of Skin Cancer

Edited by Sajjad Rajpar & Jerry Marsden
Sandwell & West Birmingham NHS Trust; Selly Oak Hospital, Birmingham

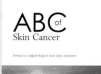

- A new, highly illustrated, concise, factual, and practical overview of skin cancers and pre-cancerous lesions
- Focuses on diagnosis, differential diagnosis, common pitfalls, and outlines best practice management in primary care
- In line with the latest NICE guidelines in the UK, places the emphasis on the pivotal role that GPs play in the screening, diagnosis and referral of skin cancers and pre-cancerous lesions
- Also includes chapters on non-surgical treatment and prevention

April 2008 | 9781405162197 | 80 pages | £19.99/$39.95/€24.90

ABC of Clinical Electrocardiography
SECOND EDITION

Edited by Francis Morris, William Brady & John Camm
Northern General Hospital, Sheffield; University of Virginia Health Sciences Centre, Charlottesville; St. George's University of London

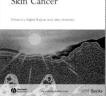

- A new edition of this practical guide to the interpretation of ECGs for the non-specialist
- The *ABC* format lends itself to clearly illustrate full 12-lead ECGs
- Sets out the main patterns seen in cardiac disorders in clinical practice, covering the fundamentals of interpretation and analysis
- Covers exercise tolerance testing and provides clear anatomical illustrations to explain key points

May 2008 | 9781405170642 | 112 pages | £26.99/$49.95/€34.90

ABC of Complementary Medicine
SECOND EDITION

Edited by Catherine Zollman, Andrew J. Vickers & Janet Richardson
General Practitioner, Bristol; Memorial Sloan-Kettering Cancer Center, New York; University of Plymouth

- This thoroughly revised and updated second edition offers an authoritative introduction to complementary therapies
- Includes the latest information on efficacy of treatments
- Places a new emphasis in patient management
- Ideal guide for primary care practitioners

June 2008 | 9781405136570 | 64 pages | £21.99/$40.95/€27.90

ABC of Eating Disorders

Edited by Jane Morris
Royal Edinburgh Hospital

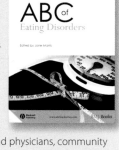

- Charts the diagnosis of different eating disorders and their management and treatment by GPs, dieticians and psychiatrists
- Examines diagnosis, management and treatment by health professionals and through self-help
- Helps primary care practitioners recognise eating disorders in young people presenting with other problems
- Supports the work of general psychiatrists and physicians, community health teams and teaching staff
- Includes medico-legal aspects of treating eating disorders and specialist referral

August 2008 | 9780727918437 | 80 pages | £19.99/$35.95/€24.90

ABC of Tubes, Drains, Lines and Frames

Edited by Adam Brooks, Peter F. Mahoney & Brian Rowlands
Queen's Medical Centre, University of Nottingham; The Royal Centre for Defence Medicine; The Royal Centre for Defence Medicine

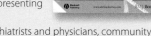

- A brand new title in the *ABC* series
- A full-colour, practical guide to the key issues involved in the assessment and management of surgical adjuncts
- Covers the care of post-operative patients in primary care
- Highlights common pitfalls and includes "trouble shooting" sections

October 2008 | 9781405160148 | 88 pages | £19.99/$35.95/€24.90

ABC of Headache

Edited by Anne MacGregor & Alison Frith
Both The City of London Migraine Clinic

- Uses real case histories to guide the reader through symptoms to diagnosis and management or, where relevant, to specialist referral
- A highly illustrated, informative and practical source of knowledge and offers links to further information and resources
- An essential guide for healthcare professionals, at all levels of training, looking for possible causes of presenting symptoms of headache

October 2008 | 9781405170666 | 88 pages | £19.99/$35.95/€24.90

ALSO AVAILABLE

ABC of Adolescence
Russell Viner
2005 | 9780727915740 | 56 pages | £19.99/$35.95/€24.90

ABC of Aids, 5th Edition
Michael W. Adler
2001 | 9780727915030 | 128 pages | £24.99/$46.95/€32.90

ABC of Alcohol, 4th Edition
Alexander Paton & Robin Touquet
2005 | 9780727918147 | 72 pages | £19.99/$35.95/€24.90

ABC of Allergies
Stephen R. Durham
1998 | 9780727912367 | 65 pages | £24.99/$44.95/€32.90

ABC of Antenatal Care, 4th Edition
Geoffrey Chamberlain & Margery Morgan
2002 | 9780727916921 | 92 pages | £22.99/$41.95/€29.90

ABC of Antithrombotic Therapy
Gregory Y.H. Lip & Andrew D. Blann
2003 | 9780727917713 | 67 pages | £19.99/$35.95/€24.90

ABC of Asthma, 5th Edition
John Rees & Dipak Kanabar
2005 | 9780727918604 | 80 pages | £24.99/$44.95/€32.90

ABC of Brainstem Death, 2nd Edition
Christopher Pallis & D.H. Harley
1996 | 9780727902450 | 55 pages | £25.99/$46.95/€32.90

ABC of Breast Diseases, 3rd Edition
J. Michael Dixon
2005 | 9780727918284 | 120 pages | £27.99/$50.95/€34.90

ABC of Burns
Shehan Hettiaratchy, Remo Papini & Peter Dziewulski
2004 | 9780727917874 | 56 pages | £19.99/$35.95/€24.90

ABC of Child Protection, 4th Edition
Sir Roy Meadow, Jacqueline Mok & Donna Rosenberg
2007 | 9780727918178 | 120 pages | £27.99/$50.95/€34.90

ABC of Clinical Genetics, 3rd Edition
Helen M. Kingston
2002 | 9780727916273 | 120 pages | £25.99/$47.95/€32.90

ABC of Clinical Haematology, 3rd Edition
Drew Provan
2007 | 9781405153539 | 112 pages | £27.99/$50.95/€34.90

ABC of Colorectal Cancer
David Kerr, Annie Young & Richard Hobbs
2001 | 9780727915269 | 39 pages | £19.99/$35.95/€24.90

ABC of Colorectal Diseases, 2nd Edition
David Jones
1998 | 9780727911056 | 110 pages | £27.99/$50.95/€34.90

ABC of Conflict and Disaster
Anthony Redmond, Peter F. Mahoney, James Ryan, Cara Macnab & Lord David Owen
2005 | 9780727917263 | 80 pages | £19.99/$35.95/€24.90

ABC of COPD
Graeme P. Currie
2006 | 9781405147118 | 48 pages | £19.99/$35.95/€24.90

ABC of Diabetes, 5th Edition
Peter J. Watkins
2002 | 9780727916938 | 108 pages | £27.99/$50.95/€34.90

ABC of Ear, Nose and Throat, 5th Edition
Harold S. Ludman & Patrick Bradley
2007 | 9781405136563 | 120 pages | £27.99/$50.95/€34.90

ABC of Emergency Radiology, 2nd Edition
Otto Chan
2007 | 9780727915283 | 144 pages | £29.99/$53.95/€37.90

ABC of Eyes, 4th Edition
Peng T. Khaw, Peter Shah & Andrew R. Elkington
2004 | 9780727916594 | 104 pages | £25.99/$46.95/€32.90

ABC of Health Informatics
Frank Sullivan & Jeremy Wyatt
2006 | 9780727918505 | 56 pages | £19.99/$35.95/€24.90

ABC of Heart Failure, 2nd Edition
Russell C. Davis, Michael K. Davies & Gregory Y.H. Lip
2006 | 9780727916440 | 72 pages | £19.99/$35.95/€24.90

ABC of Hypertension, 5th Edition
Gareth Beevers, Gregory Y.H. Lip & Eoin O'Brien
2007 | 9781405130615 | 88 pages | £24.99/$44.95/€32.90

ABC of Intensive Care
Mervyn Singer & Ian Grant
1999 | 9780727914361 | 64 pages | £17.99/$31.95/€24.90

ABC of Interventional Cardiology
Ever D. Grech
2003 | 9780727915467 | 51 pages | £19.99/$35.95/€24.90

ABC of Kidney Disease
David Goldsmith, Satishkumar Abeythunge Jayawardene & Penny Ackland
2007 | 9781405136754 | 96 pages | £26.99/$49.95/€34.90

ABC of Labour Care
Geoffrey Chamberlain, Philip Steer & Luke Zander
1999 | 9780727914156 | 60 pages | £18.99/$33.95/€24.90

ABC of Learning and Teaching in Medicine
Peter Cantillon, Linda Hutchinson & Diana Wood
2003 | 9780727916785 | 64 pages | £18.99/$33.95/€24.90

ABC of Liver, Pancreas and Gall Bladder
Ian Beckingham
2001 | 9780727915313 | 64 pages | £18.99/$33.95/€24.90

ABC of Major Trauma, 3rd Edition
Peter Driscoll, David Skinner & Richard Earlam
1999 | 9780727913784 | 192 pages | £24.99/$46.95/€32.90

ABC of Mental Health
Teifion Davies & T.K.J. Craig
1998 | 9780727912206 | 120 pages | £27.99/$50.95/€34.90

ABC of Monitoring Drug Therapy
Jeffrey Aronson, M. Hardman & D. J. M. Reynolds
1993 | 9780727907912 | 46 pages | £19.99/$35.95/€24.90

ABC of Nutrition, 4th Edition
A. Stewart Truswell
2003 | 9780727916648 | 152 pages | £25.99/$46.95/€32.90

ABC of Obesity
Naveed Sattar & Mike Lean
2007 | 9781405136747 | 64 pages | £19.99/$33.95/€24.90

ABC of Occupational and Environmental Medicine, 2nd Edition
David Snashall & Dipti Patel
2003 | 9780727916112 | 124 pages | £27.99/$50.95/€34.90

ABC of One To Seven, 4th Edition
Bernard Valman
1999 | 9780727912329 | 156 pages | £27.99/$50.95/€34.90

ABC of Oral Health
Crispian Scully
2000 | 9780727915511 | 41 pages | £18.99/$33.95/€24.90

ABC of Palliative Care, 2nd Edition
Marie Fallon & Geoffrey Hanks
2006 | 9781405130790 | 96 pages | £23.99/$44.95/€29.90

ABC of Patient Safety
John Sandars & Gary Cook
2007 | 9781405156929 | 64 pages | £22.99/$40.95/€29.90

ABC of Preterm Birth
William McGuire & Peter Fowlie
2005 | 9780727917638 | 56 pages | £19.99/$35.95/€24.90

ABC of Psychological Medicine
Richard Mayou, Michael Sharpe & Alan Carson
2003 | 9780727915566 | 72 pages | £19.99/$35.95/€24.90

ABC of Resuscitation, 5th Edition
Michael Colquhoun, Anthony Handley & T.R. Evans
2003 | 9780727916693 | 111 pages | £27.99/$50.95/€34.90

ABC of Rheumatology, 3rd Edition
Michael L. Snaith
2004 | 9780727916884 | 136 pages | £25.99/$46.95/€32.90

ABC of Sexual Health, 2nd Edition
John Tomlinson
2004 | 9780727917591 | 96 pages | £24.99/$44.95/€32.90

ABC of Sexually Transmitted Infections, 5th Edition
Michael W. Adler, Frances Cowan, Patrick French, Helen Mitchell & John Richens
2004 | 9780727917614 | 104 pages | £24.99/$46.95/€32.90

ABC of Smoking Cessation
John Britton
2004 | 9780727918185 | 56 pages | £17.99/$33.95/€22.90

ABC of Sports and Exercise Medicine, 3rd Edition
Gregory Whyte, Mark Harries & Clyde Williams
2005 | 9780727918130 | 136 pages | £27.99/$53.95/€34.90

ABC of Subfertility
Peter Braude & Alison Taylor
2004 | 9780727915344 | 64 pages | £18.99/$33.95/€24.90

ABC of the Upper Gastrointestinal Tract
Robert Logan, Adam Harris, J.J. Misiewicz & J.H. Baron
2002 | 9780727912664 | 54 pages | £19.99/$35.95/€24.90

ABC of Urology, 2nd Edition
Chris Dawson & Hugh N. Whitfield
2006 | 9781405139595 | 64 pages | £21.99/$40.95/€27.90

ABC of Wound Healing
Joseph E. Grey & Keith G. Harding
2006 | 9780727916952 | 56 pages | £19.99/$35.95/€24.90

To order call **0800 243407** (UK only) or **+44 1243 843294** (from overseas), email **cs-books@wiley.co.uk** or visit **www.wiley.com**